Law and Professional Issues in Nursing

Richard Griffith and Cassam Tengnah

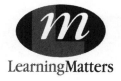

LearningMatters

First published in 2008 by Learning Matters Ltd
Reprinted in 2009

British Library Cataloguing in Publication Data
A CIP record for this book is available from the British Library
ISBN: 978 1 84445 160 9

Cover design by Topics – The Creative Partnership
Text design by Code 5 Design Associates Ltd
Project Management by Diana Chambers
Typeset by Kelly Gray
Printed and bound in Great Britain by TJ International Ltd, Padstow, Cornwall

Learning Matters Ltd
33 Southernhay East
Exeter EX1 1NX
Tel: 01392 215560
E-mail: info@learningmatters.co.uk
www.learningmatters.co.uk

**7 – DAY
LOAN**

nal

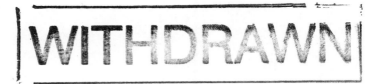

Series Editor: Shirley Bach

Transforming Nursing Practice – titles in the series

Law and Professional Issues in Nursing	ISBN 978 1 84445 160 9
Nursing and Working with Other People	ISBN 978 1 84445 161 6
Nursing in Contemporary Healthcare Practice	ISBN 978 1 84445 159 3

To order, contact our distributor: BEBC Distribution, Albion Close, Parkstone, Poole, BH12 3LL. Telephone: 0845 230 9000, email: **learningmatters@bebc.co.uk**. You can also find more information on each of these titles and our other learning resources at **www.learningmatters.co.uk**

Contents

Foreword

Here is a text that will provide you with excellent guidance for your years as a student and as a qualified practitioner. The authors have brought together in a sensible format all you need to know about the law and how it protects and guides us for safe practice. People have different reactions to laws. Some see them as a protection for themselves, and others, against harm. Others see them as barriers or constraints hidden within dense levels of bureaucracy. Another view is that they are a baffling labyrinth of unfamiliar terms that date back to archaic times and represented by a medieval dress code – picture the lawyer in gown and wig! After reading this book you will see that laws provide the conditions from which we can pursue our professional and personal lives in a manner that safeguards our patients and those for whom we care.

In the text there is an emphasis on the law, but it is grounded in the principles of patient rights. It is this ethos that, in turn, shapes how we manage sometimes difficult moral and ethical dilemmas, always with a view to practising within the principles of the NMC *Professional Code of Conduct*. There are very detailed explanations of concepts such as accountability, responsibility, discrimination, disability and equality. You will find chapters dedicated to mental health, and children's and human rights. Difficult issues such as gaining consent from vulnerable groups are explained with examples to illustrate how the laws can be understood and applied.

The concluding chapters on record keeping, confidentiality, and health and safety provide up-to-date information on aspects of professional care that are integral to our activities. Yet they are often so ingrained that we neglect the significance of the laws that are designed to protect our patients and provide professional safeguards. These chapters provide essential, practical guidance to achieve good practice and meet legal requirements.

In each chapter the relevant NMC *Standards of Proficiency* are stated and will be a feature of the Transforming Nursing Practice series. This ensures that nursing students will see exactly how the information in the book relates to achieving their competencies and be ready to practise in the contemporary world of nursing we know today.

Shirley Bach
Series Editor

Table of cases

A v United Kingdom [1998] 2 FLR 959.
A&D v B&E [2003] EWHC 1376 (FAM).
Airedale NHS Trust v Bland [1993] AC 789.
Archibald v Fife Council [2004] UKHL 32.
Association X v United Kingdom (7154/75) (1978) European Commission on Human Rights.
Attorney General v Guardian Newspapers Ltd [1987] 1 WLR 1248.
Attorney General v Mulholland [1963] 2 QB 477.
B v B (A Minor) (Residence Order) [1992] 2 FLR 327.
B v B (Minors) (Residence and Care Disputes) [1994] 2 FLR 489.
B v Croydon HA [1995] 2 WLR 294.
B v United Kingdom (36536/02) [2005] All ER D 63.
Barnado v McHugh [1891] AC 388 (CA).
Barnett v Chelsea and Kensington Hospital Management Committee [1969] 1 QB 428
    (QBD).
Bayliss v Blagg and Another (1954) 1 BMJ 709.
Blyth v Birmingham Waterworks (1856) 11 Exch. 781.
Blyth v Bloomsbury HA [1993] 4 Med LR 151.
Bolam v Friern HMC [1957] 1 WLR 582.
Bolitho v City and Hackney HA [1998] AC 232.
Bolton v Stone [1951] AC 850.
British Home Stores Ltd v Burchell [1980] ICR 303 (EAT).
C and B (Children) (Care Order:Future Harm) [2000] 2 FCR 614.
C v C [1946] 1 All ER 562.
Camden LBC v R (A Minor) (Blood Transfusion) [1993] 2 FLR 757.
Caparo Industries Plc v Dickman [1992] 2 AC 605 (HL).
Centre for Reproductive Medicine v U [2002] EWCA Civ 565.
Chester v Afshar [2002] EWCA 724.
Ciarlariello v Schacter [1991] 2 Med. LR 391.
Cornelius v De Taranto [2001] EWCA Civ 1511.
Council for the Regulation of Health Care Professionals v (1) The Nursing and Midwifery
    Council (2) Steven Truscott [2004] EWCA Civ 1356.
Cruickshank v VAW Motorcast Ltd [2002] ICR 729.
D v National Society for the Prevention of Cruelty to Children [1977] 2 WLR 201.
D v United Kingdom [1997] 24 EHRR 423.
Deacon v McVicar (1984) (Unreported Queens Bench Division 7th June).
Devi v West Midlands RHA [1981] EWHC 1980.
Dewen v Barnet Healthcare Trust and Barnet London Borough Council [2000] 2 FLR 848.

Table of statutes

Table of secondary legislation

Health and Safety (First Aid) Regulations 1981 (1981/917).
United Nations (1989) Convention on the Rights of the Child adopted under General
    Assembly Resolution 44/25.
Health and Safety (Display Screen Equipment) Regulations 1992 (1992/2792).
Manual Handling Operations Regulations 1992 (1992/2793).
Personal Protective Equipment at Work Regulations 1992 (1992/2966).
Workplace (Health, Safety and Welfare) Regulations 1992 (1992/3004).
Reporting of Injuries, Diseases and Dangerous Occurrences Regulations 1995
    (1995/3163).
Health and Safety (Consultation with Employees) Regulations 1996 (1996/1513).
Health and Safety (Safety Signs and Signals) Regulations 1996 (1996/0341).
Fire Precautions (Workplaces) Regulations 1997 (1997/1840).
Safety Representatives and Safety Committee Regulations 1977 (1997/500).
Provision and Use of Work Equipment Regulations 1998 (1998/2306).
Health Service Commissioner (1999) *Inappropriate Response to Deterioration in the
    Condition of a Patient over the Weekend against Hastings and Rother NHS Trust –
    Case No. E.2291/98–99.*
Management of Health and Safety at Work Regulations 1999 (SI 1999/3242).
Control of Substances Hazardous to Health Regulations 2002 (SI 2002/2677).
Health Service (Control of Patient Information) Regulations 2002 (SI 2002/1438).
Nursing and Midwifery Order 2001 (SI 2002/253).
Medicines for Human Use (Clinical Trials) Regulations 2004 (SI 2004/1031).
Hazardous Waste (England and Wales)Regulations 2005 (SI 2005/894).
Medicines for Human Use (Prescribing) (Miscellaneous Amendments) Order 2006
    (SI 2006/915).
Mental Health (Nurses) (England) Order 2008 (SI 2008/1207).

Introduction

The position of the patient in health and social care is more legalised now than ever before. A wide range of laws regulate the relationship between the nurse and patient. It is essential that as a nurse you have a sound working knowledge of the legislation and policies that govern your practice.

These requirements are reflected in the Nursing and Midwifery Council's Standards of Proficiency for entry onto the register. As a student nurse you must achieve these proficiencies in order to become a registered nurse.

Standard 7 of the proficiencies for pre-registration education concerns the standards for professional and ethical practice. It highlights the legal and professional principles that you must know in order to practice safely, effectively and within the law.

This book focuses on the legal and professional issues that you as a student nurse must understand and apply in order to demonstrate that you are competent to enter your chosen branch programme. It reflects the requirements of the Nursing and Midwifery Council updated *Code: Standards of performance, ethics and nurses and midwives* that was introduced in May 2008. The book also includes the amendments to mental health law introduced by the Mental Health Act 2007.

Chapter 1 introduces you to the legal system and a framework for ethical decision making in nursing. Chapter 2 describes how professional practice as a registered nurse is regulated by the law through the concept of accountability. The two chapters cover fundamental topics that underpin a registered nurse's relationship with their patients, profession and society, making them essential reading for you and all student nurses.

The remaining chapters relate to specific competencies set by the Nursing and Midwifery Council for entry onto the branch programme. The legal and professional principles considered in these chapters will guide you through the complex legal problems you are likely to encounter in your career as a registered nurse. For example, you will see how a legal standard of care is imposed on you through the law of negligence; how laws such as the Human Rights Act 1998, Mental Health Act 1983 and Mental Capacity Act 2005 protect vulnerable adults, and how the Children Act 1989 safeguards children.

You are given the opportunity to apply the laws discussed in these chapters to your own practice through guided activities designed to consolidate your knowledge and assist you with assignment preparation and writing. Where appropriate, a brief outline answer to the questions is given at the end of each chapter to help you.

Chapter 1, 'Introduction to law and ethics in nursing' emphasises that law is fundamental to the study of nursing and underpins your relationship with the profession and with your patients. It is essential that as a student nurse you are able to understand and critically reflect on legal issues relevant to nursing practice.

The law informs nursing at every stage and it is essential that you understand and are able to reflect critically on the legal issues relevant to nursing practice.

The standards of the profession and its regulatory body, the Nursing and Midwifery Council, are derived from the law and underpinned by fundamental ethical principles as reflected in the Nursing and Midwifery Council's *Code: Standards of conduct, performance and ethics for nurses and midwives* (NMC, 2008).

A principle based approach to ethical decision making is introduced in the chapter to assist you to apply the law appropriately, effectively and within the requirements of your professional code.

In Chapter 2, 'Accountability', we discuss how this fundamental concept is crucial to the protection of the public and individual patients, particularly where they are vulnerable adults or children. It is essential that the term is clearly understood by nurses as it is the means by which the law imposes standards and boundaries on professional practice. This chapter considers how the law creates four spheres of accountability that are imposed on registered nurses and the standard of conduct each requires. Accountability is the concept that underpins the legal and professional issues that apply to nursing.

Chapter 3, 'Equality and human rights', explains how nursing must be practised with respect for the rights and freedoms of others and a recognition of the needs of the diverse cultures that make up the population of the United Kingdom. This chapter considers how the law promotes equality and human rights in the modern health service and emphasises that, as a registered nurse, you will have a legal duty to ensure that you do not discriminate on the grounds of race or disability. The chapter also considers the role of human rights in healthcare and in particular discusses the dual obligation on a registered nurse to protect vulnerable adults and children by championing their human rights and ensuring that they do not practise in a way that breaches human rights.

Chapter 4, 'Consent to treatment', examines how nursing is very much a hands-on, interactive profession and nurses regularly need to touch their patients in order to examine them or provide care and treatment. Touching a person without consent is generally unlawful and will amount to a trespass to the person or, more rarely, a criminal assault.

This chapter considers how the law promotes the autonomy of an adult patient and what constitutes a real consent. It then discusses how the provisions of the Mental Capacity Act 2005 protects vulnerable adults and young persons by regulating how decisions are made for those who lack capacity to make a decision about care and treatment themselves.

In Chapter 5, 'Mental Health', we look at how the position of the patient with mental health problems is now regulated by a range of legislation that seeks to protect those adults and children considered to be vulnerable in our society. This chapter considers the key provisions of the Mental Health Act 1983 as amended by the Mental Health Act 2007, and the strong body of case law that has developed from it dealing with fundamental issues of liberty, autonomy and respect. The chapter emphasises that when caring for a person with mental health problems it is essential that as a nurse you not only apply the requirements of the legislation accurately but do so ethically and with due regard for the rights of the vulnerable patients in your care.

Chapter 6, 'Consent and children', focuses on the issue of consent in relation to children and follows the law as it changes to take account of the development of the child to adulthood. Consent is considered in relation to a child of tender years, a Gillick competent child and the 16- and 17-year-old child.

Chapter 7, 'Safeguarding children', examines the way in which nurses have a key role in the identification of children who may have been abused or who are at risk of abuse.

They are also well placed to recognise when parents or other adults have problems that might affect their capacity to fulfil their roles with children safely. Nurses must have a sound working knowledge of the Children Acts of 1989 and 2004 and know when to refer a child for help as a 'child in need' and how to act on concerns that a child is at risk of significant harm through abuse or neglect.

Chapter 8, 'Negligence', examines how the law imposes a standard of care on nurses, requiring them to be careful when caring for patients. Failing to meet that standard and harming a patient means the nurse will be accountable for their carelessness through the law of negligence. This chapter considers the elements of a negligence action and the extent of a nurse's duty of care towards their patients. It goes on to discuss negligence as a criminal act through a discussion of the offence of gross negligence manslaughter.

Chapter 9, 'Recordkeeping', considers the importance of recordkeeping and how nurses should write records to ensure that the legal requirements are met. By drawing on case law it also highlights the consequences for nurses of failing to meet those requirements.

Chapter 10, 'Confidentiality', looks at how maintaining the confidentiality of a patient's health information is a fundamental element of professional conduct and ethical practice for all registered nurses. The relationship between nurse and patient is essential for proper assessment and care that is largely based on a patient's personal history of their health problem. Patients pass on sensitive information in confidence and expect you to respect their privacy by ensuring the confidentiality of the information they give.

Chapter 11, 'Health and safety' considers the legal duties imposed on nurses under the Health and Safety at Work Act 1974 and its regulations. It goes on to discuss the four main causes of accidents in the NHS and how the health and safety of employees and patients can be safeguarded.

Chapter 1

Introduction to law and ethics in nursing

NMC Standards of Proficiency

This chapter will address the following NMC *Standards of Proficiency* and *Outcomes to be achieved for entry to the branch programme.*

Practise in accordance with an ethical and legal framework which ensures the primacy of patient and client interest and well-being and respects confidentiality.

Outcomes to be achieved for entry to the branch programme:
Demonstrate an awareness of, and apply ethical principles to, nursing practice:

- identify ethical issues in day to day practice.

Chapter aims

By the end of this chapter you will be able to:

- identify primary and secondary sources of legal material;
- outline the role of statutes in law;
- state the role of precedent at common law;
- describe the terms 'morals' and 'ethics';
- outline the principle-based approach;
- explain how the principle-based approach can be used when considering a moral problem relating to practice.

Introduction

A book on legal and professional issues in nursing may seem an unusual collection of topics for a course of study that will largely focus on meeting the needs of individuals with various health problems. Why is it necessary for you to study law when you want to devote your time to the study of nursing and caring for patients?

The reality is that law is now fundamental to the study of nursing and underpins your relationship with the profession and with your patients. The law informs nursing at every stage and it is essential that you understand and are able to critically reflect on the legal issues relevant to nursing practice.

When you take on the care of a patient you undertake a duty of care towards that person not to harm them in accordance with the law of negligence. The care and treatment you provide will be based on the law of consent and the informed and freely given permission of the patient will be a prerequisite to any lawful treatment. The legal principles of confidentiality and negligence will regulate the relationship between you and the patient while they are in your care.

The standards of the profession and its regulatory body, the Nursing and Midwifery Council (NMC), are derived from the fundamental ethical principles of respect for autonomy, ensuring that a nurse's actions are for the benefit of your patients through the principle of beneficence, doing no harm to patients by ensuring non-maleficence and being fair, or just dealing with patients and the wider community so that you reflect the principle of justice. These principles largely underpin the law relating to healthcare and the standards of conduct, performance and ethics required of you by the NMC in *The Code: Standards of conduct, performance and ethics for nurses* and *midwives* (NMC, 2008).

Activity 1.1

The Code

The standards imposed on registered nurses by the Nursing and Midwifery Council are contained in *The Code: Standards of conduct, performance and ethics for nurses and midwives* (NMC, 2008).

Read the *Code* which can be downloaded from the NMC website at www.nmc-uk.org, and identify the standards that apply to:

* your relationship with patients;
* your relationship with colleagues;
* your relationship with the profession;
* your relationship with society generally.

The *Code* highlights how the law and legal system applies to the nursing profession. Keep it with you as you work through this book.

The accountable practitioner

As a registered nurse you will be legally and professionally accountable for your actions, irrespective of whether you are following the instruction of another or using your own initiative. Healthcare litigation is growing and patients are increasingly prepared to assert their legal rights. Compensation payments in the National Health Service (NHS) are currently running at some £500 million a year (NHS Litigation Authority, 2007).

It is perhaps little wonder, therefore, that the NMC insists that student nurses are able to practise in accordance with an ethical and legal framework that ensures the primacy of patient and client interest (NMC, 2004c).

A thorough and critical appreciation of the legal, ethical and professional issues affecting nursing practice is essential if you are to develop the professional awareness necessary to satisfy the NMC that you are an accountable practitioner, competent to practise as a registered nurse.

Defining law

Activity 1.2

The law

Before reading on, think about the laws you are aware of and what their role is; then write down what you believe the term law means.
Now read the following for further guidance.

A typical dictionary would define law as:

a rule enacted or customary in a community and recognised as commanding or forbidding certain actions;

or

a body of such rules.

A key characteristic of law is that it is perceived as binding upon the community. The English word 'law' is derived from the Old Norse meaning 'laid down' or 'fixed'. The definition suggests that law is made up of rules, but is it the case that all rules have legal force?

Activity 1.3

Normative and positive rules

Consider the following rules – which of these rules do you think are laws?

- Honour your mother and father.
- Do not steal.
- Be truthful in all circumstances.
- Do not kill other people.
- Rescue your neighbour's drowning child.
- Register a child's birth.
- Do not park on double yellow lines.

See below for an explanation of the rules.

Positive rules

Positive rules impose a legal obligation to do or refrain from doing something. If a positive rule is breached, a sanction may be imposed for breaking the law.

Normative rules

Normative rules set out what a person should do, or what they should refrain from doing. Note the word *should* – the individual is not compelled to abide by normative rules, they simply ought to. Normative rules are based on values that highlight a desired form of conduct but they do not carry legal force.

In the last activity the positive rules were:

- Do not kill other people – it is a common law offence to kill other people; that is the offence of murder.
- Do not park on double yellow lines – parking on double yellow lines constitutes a road traffic offence.
- Do not steal – stealing is an offence under the Theft Act 1968.
- Register a child's birth – an example of the law requiring a particular action, in this case under the Birth and Deaths Registration Act 1875.

The normative rules were:

- Honour your mother and father – this is established through religious teachings and reflects the fifth commandment of the Ten Commandments. It is not a requirement of the law in the UK.
- Be truthful in all circumstances – veracity is a moral or ethical issue. The need to be truthful in law occurs in specific circumstances such as when giving evidence under oath.
- Rescue your neighbour's drowning child – there is generally no duty of simple rescue in the UK. If you had a professional duty such as being a lifeguard at a swimming pool, you would be legally obliged to rescue the child.

In some cases the law requires that a person take action, for example the requirement that a child's birth be registered. However, in most cases the law requires a person to refrain from doing something, for example from killing others, parking on double yellow lines or stealing.

Relevance to healthcare

In healthcare we see a drawing together of normative and positive rules. The law imposes a minimum standard of acceptable care and behaviour on you as a registered nurse. Patients, however, deserve the highest possible standard of care and behaviour, so the health and social care organisation where you work and the profession, through *The Code* (2008), will require a standard that is higher than the law expects.

The Code is underpinned by a shared set of values common to all United Kingdom (UK) healthcare regulatory bodies. In a clear drawing together of both normative and positive rules, it requires that as a registered nurse you:

- respect the patient or client as an individual;
- obtain consent before you give any treatment or care;
- protect confidential information;
- cooperate with others in the team;
- maintain your professional knowledge and competence;
- be trustworthy;
- act to identify and minimise risk to patients and clients.

During your training as a student nurse you will be expected to live up to the standards of the Nursing and Midwifery Council's *Code* and the law and professional issues that underpin them. Higher Education institutions have Fitness to Practice panels where students who are accused of falling below the standards required of them are held to account. The decisions of the panels are based on the fitness to practice guidance espoused by the *Code*.

Criminal and civil law

The same unlawful action can be dealt with in different ways by the law. For example, touching a person without permission, that is without consent, can be both a crime and a *tort* – a civil wrong.

The crime would be charged under the Offences Against the Person Act 1861. This very old statute is still very much in force today and forbids many forms of unlawful touching, such as actual bodily harm (section 47), wounding (sections 18 and 20), or even procuring a miscarriage (section 58). A crime is an act that is capable of being followed by criminal proceedings and with an outcome, an acquittal or a conviction that is criminal in nature.

Unlawful touching can also be pursued through the civil courts as the tort of trespass to the person. The law of tort is primarily concerned with providing a remedy, by way of compensation, to persons who have been harmed by the conduct of others.

The nature of law

From our discussion of the law we can define law as:

> A rule of human conduct imposed upon and enforced among the members of a given state.

Two ideas underpin this notion of the law:

- **order**, in the sense that there is a method or legal system that underpins the creation and implementation of the law; and
- **compulsion**, or the enforcement of obedience to the rules that are laid down by the law.

Sources of legal material

In your study of the law as it applies to healthcare and nursing, you will use a range of primary and secondary sources of law to inform your practice and your studies. Figure 1.1 highlights the typical sources of primary and secondary legal material that you can use in your studies.

Sources of primary legal material

Although there are many textbooks and periodicals that discuss legal issues in nursing, it is best whenever possible to study the primary legal material as well. This will give you a detailed understanding of the law as it relates to nursing.

There are three major sources of primary legal material, as follows.

Legislation
- Acts of Parliament that may also be referred to as Statute law or *lex scripta* (written law).
- Secondary legislation:
  - Statutory instruments, which are also known as delegated legislation and subordinate legislation.

Judicial decisions
These are decisions from cases decided in court, and are also known as the common law or *lex non scripta* (unwritten law from judges).

Figure 1.1: Sources of legal material.

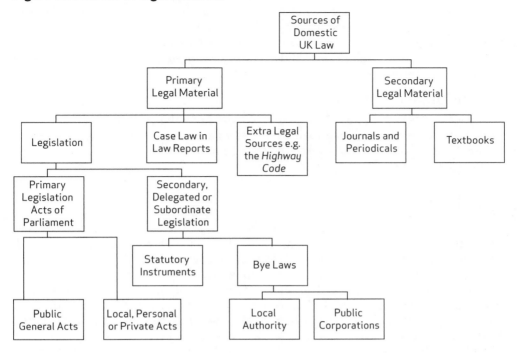

European Community and human rights law

Parliament has allowed these areas to be sources of law by incorporating them through Acts of Parliament (The European Community Act 1972 and the Human Rights Act 1998).

Royal Prerogative

The Royal Prerogative used to be the main source of law before the development of the parliamentary system in the UK. It now describes the powers, handed down direct from monarchs to ministers over many years, that allow governments, among other things, to go to war, regulate the Civil Service, issue passports and grant honours, all without any need for approval from Parliament. As these powers have been handed down over many centuries new powers cannot be created.

When having to consider a novel dispute or how to apply an ancient law to a modern situation, judges will often take account of extra legal sources to assist them, such as the following.

Received wisdom

- Legal writers: The law is extensively analysed and tested by academics and practitioners, and judges often resort to such analysis to assist them when having to decide a novel or complex case.
- Public opinion: In *Gillick v West Norfolk and Wisbech AHA* [1986], a case concerning the lawfulness of giving contraceptive treatment to girls under the age of 16, the House of Lords heard an appeal from the Court of Appeal, which had made a decision relying on a seventeenth-century precedent. Lord Scarman, in his opinion, said that part of the court's function was to reflect public opinion and to bring the law kicking and screaming into the twentieth century.

Codes and best practice

Judges will also refer to extra legal sources of law that bring together normative and positive rules and signal best practice in a particular area. For example, where a judge has to decide if a nurse's conduct is acceptable, then he or she will refer to the NMC's *Code* (2008). In a road traffic case the judge will refer to the *Highway Code*. These sources are only ever persuasive on a judge, who is not bound by them.

Laws from other countries

Where an issue arises that has never been considered by the courts, then judges may consider how the matter was dealt with in other legal systems. The laws and cases of other jurisdictions can be considered by the court, but again they can only be a source of persuasion and are never binding on the court.

Legislation

The UK is a parliamentary democracy and the laws of the country are created and amended through the Queen in Parliament. That is, a new law or bill is considered, debated and scrutinised by the elected House of Commons and appointed House of Lords before receiving Royal Assent and becoming an Act of Parliament.

The Acts you are concerned with in your studies are *public general Acts*. These apply to classes or sub-classes of people. For example, the Mental Health Act 1983 concerns the care and treatment of people with mental disorder; the Children Act 1989 concerns the welfare of children.

You will not be concerned with *private Acts*, which have a much narrower application and concern local issues and persons. For example, a private Act of Parliament, the Valerie Mary Hill and Alan Monk (Marriage Enabling) Act 1985, had to be passed to allow a man to marry his ex-wife's mother (his mother-in-law) – an action generally forbidden by the Marriage Act 1960.

The function of Acts

Acts of Parliament are generally created to fulfil one of five main purposes.

Revision of substantive rules of law

The laws of the UK need to be kept up to date and Acts are created to modernise existing law in order to bring it into line with modern society. A body known as the Law Commission keeps law under review and makes suggestions for reform. These are not always acted upon in a timely manner, however. For example, a Law Commission report (Law Commission, 1993) into decision making for incapable adults, submitted in 1993, eventually resulted in the Mental Capacity Act 2005.

Consolidation of Acts

Laws build up in a piecemeal fashion over many years and there is often a need to consolidate different parts of a law into one Act of Parliament. For example, the Health and Safety at Work etc. Act 1974 consolidated several other Acts concerning safety in the workplace, including the Mines and Quarries Act 1954, the Agriculture (Safety, Health and Welfare Provisions) Act 1956, the Factories Act 1961, the Offices, Shops and Railway Premises Act 1963, The Nuclear Installations Act 1965 and the Mines and Quarries (Tips) Act 1969.

Codification

Codification means putting a rule of the common law into statute law. Where a decision in a case is considered fundamental or very important, Parliament will codify it by making the rule part of an Act. For example in *R v Bourne* [1939], a surgeon was acquitted of procuring a miscarriage by abortion when a jury decided that doing so to preserve the mental and physical health of the mother was lawful. When the Abortion Act 1967 was enacted, Parliament codified that decision under section 1(1) of the 1967 Act.

Collection of revenue

Taxation is a function of Acts. Each year the Government presents its budget to Parliament, which allows the raising of revenue through taxation.

Social legislation

This is a broad category that covers the many facets of running the country. It is the main area of party political differences and the main source of debate in Parliament.

How a bill becomes an Act of Parliament

There are many stages that a bill has to go through before it can become an Act of Parliament (see Figure 1.2).

Figure 1.2: Stages of a bill.

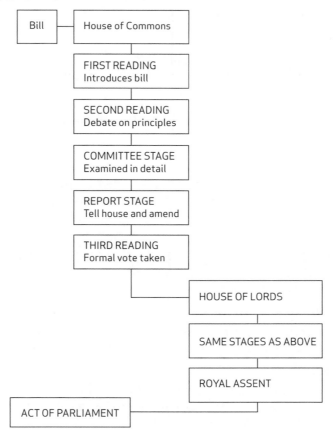

Manifesto

All political parties have a manifesto, which is their promise to the electorate of the actions they will take and the laws they will pass if they become the Government. It is these promises that persuade us to vote for a party.

Not all such promises become law, because when a party takes office they are supplied with detailed information by senior civil servants and may discover that the reforms are not realistic, or are too expensive.

Other laws enacted during a Government's term of office will be a reaction to an event, such as a war, or a ruling by the courts. In 2005, a man argued that having to ask for a private Act to be allowed to marry his mother-in-law was a violation of his human rights and the Government was forced to change the law to bring it into line with the Human Rights Act 1998 (*B v United Kingdom (36536/02)* [2005]).

Queen's Speech

The Queen's Speech at the State Opening of Parliament in November announces the main bills constituting the Government's legislative programme. The Government actually writes the speech for the Queen to read.

Green Papers

Green Papers – or Command Papers – are consultation papers that seek comments from the public. The importance of consultation was seen when Tony Blair attempted to abolish the role of the Lord Chancellor without first consulting anyone. He then discovered that this could not happen without first changing over 500 statutes that referred to the functions of the Lord Chancellor.

White Papers

Following the Green Paper, the Government will present to Parliament a White Paper, which is a statement of policy and contains definite proposals for legislation.

Drafting

After consultation, Parliamentary Counsel (Draftsmen) will draft a bill into the form of words necessary for a bill.

Bills

In order to become an Act of Parliament, a bill must be passed by both Houses of Parliament and receive Royal Assent (collectively known as 'the Queen in Parliament').

First reading

The first reading of a bill involves a member reading the title of the bill. The first reading takes place without debate and is essentially an announcement that the bill has been introduced, after which copies of the bill are made available for members to read and are placed on the Parliament website.

Second reading

The second reading provides the first occasion for debate on the general principles of a bill, and then detailed discussion takes place during the committee stage.

Committee stage

When a bill has passed its second reading in the House of Commons, it is then referred to a General Committee. The Committee examines the clauses of the bill line by line, word by word, and detailed amendments are considered.

Report stage

Any amendments made during the committee stage must be approved or rejected by the whole House during the report stage, which is a detailed debate where further amendments may be moved.

Third reading

The third reading of a bill often follows on immediately after the report stage. The bill is reviewed in its final form, including amendments made at earlier stages. Then the final version of the bill is approved and passed by hand – bound in green ribbon – to the Lords. When the Lords return the bill it is bound in red ribbon.

In the House of Lords, broadly the same procedure is followed.

Once all stages have been completed the bill receives Royal Assent and becomes an Act (see Figure 1.3). The date of Royal Assent is not necessarily the date the Act comes

Figure 1.3: The first page of a public general Act, with its constituent parts labelled.

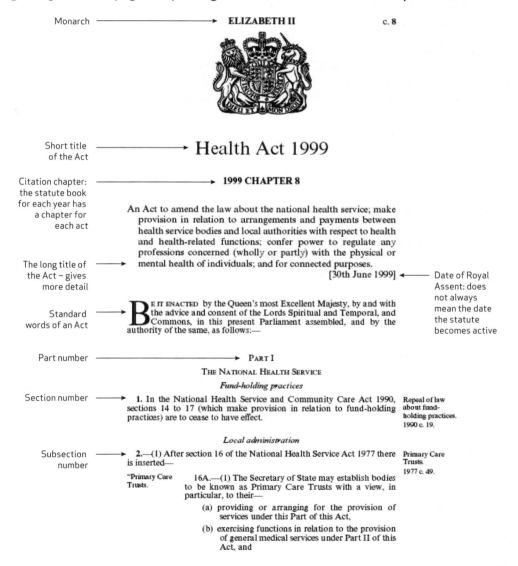

into force. Many Acts begin at a later date with the issuing of a commencement order. For example, the part of the NHS and Community Care Act 1990 that introduced the notion of the NHS Trust did not commence until 1993. The Easter Act 1928, which sets Easter on a specific date, has never come into force.

Secondary legislation

With the rigorous scrutiny that bills must undergo, only some 50 Acts are passed by Parliament each year. It is therefore not uncommon for an Act to give powers to government ministers and other public bodies to introduce secondary legislation that enables general updating of the law. Secondary legislation, also sometimes called subordinate legislation, is generally in the form of a *statutory instrument* and includes regulations and orders. For example, the Medicines for Human Use (Clinical Trials) Regulations 2004 set the requirements for testing new medicines, while the Medicines for Human Use (Prescribing) (Miscellaneous Amendments) Order 2006 introduced independent and supplementary prescribing of medicines by nurses and other health professionals.

Some 5,000 statutory instruments are approved by Parliament each year. An important statutory instrument affecting nursing is the Nursing and Midwifery Order 2001, which established the NMC. The order was created under powers given by section 60 of the Health Act 1999. Where a minister or public body acts contrary to the powers bestowed by an Act, their decision can be challenged as *ultra vires*. For example, in *London and Westcliff Properties v Minister of Housing and Local Government* [1961], a council compulsorily purchased a property, then sold it to a company at a reduced cost. The court held that this was *ultra vires*, as the Housing Act 1957 required councils to obtain the best possible price for a property.

The annotated first page of the 2001 Order is shown in Figure 1.4.

Judicial interpretation of statutes

Once an Act has completed its parliamentary stages and becomes law, the authoritative and compelling interpretation of that statute is for judges and no one else. When it comes to a dispute only the judges' views count. Governance in the UK is structured to prevent tyranny by attempting to ensure that no one person or body has an over-dominant role. The system sees three components of governance come together but as separate entities, with different roles as illustrated in Figure 1.5.

Judicial function

The role of the courts is to give force to the intention of Parliament as expressed in the words of the Act, and to make decisions between disputing parties. The courts cannot question statutes as Parliament is supreme and an Act of Parliament is our supreme source of law. Judges must apply the statute to the particular facts before them and to do this they need to interpret the words in an Act.

Parliament makes law, judges interpret and apply the law, and they have a great deal of discretion in how they do this.

Judicial decisions, the common law

The common law consists of laws that arise from cases decided by the courts. It works on a system of precedent and is often referred to in Latin as *stare decisis* or 'let the decision stand'. When a judge decides a case, he or she must refer to decisions in previous similar cases in the higher courts and keep to the rulings in those cases. If the previous case was about a similar set of facts and the same legal rules, then the current case has to be decided in the same way.

Activity 1.4

Precedent in action: the case of the snail in the ginger beer

In *Donoghue v Stevenson* [1932] two friends have a drink in a Paisley café. Mrs Donoghue has a ginger beer, which she gradually pours and drinks from an earthenware bottle from the bottom of which comes a green sludge, the remains of a decomposing snail. This causes her gastroenteritis and nervous shock, so she sues the manufacturer and the court awards her damages. The court finds that the manufacturer owes her a duty of care, which they have breached, causing her harm, because through their carelessness a snail entered the bottle in the manufacturing process.

Does precedent apply? Consider the following situations and decide whether the judge in the cases would be bound by the precedent set in the *Donoghue v Stevenson* [1932] case.

1. A woman buys a bottle of lager from Tesco. Before she opens it she sees that it contains a dead wasp. Can she sue in negligence?
2. Utilities contractors dig a hole in a pavement and mark it with an upturned sledge hammer. Most people see the hazard and avoid it but a blind man falls in and breaks a leg. Can he sue in negligence?
3. A child is eating fish fingers for school dinner when he chokes on a one-inch piece of bone that needs surgery to remove. His mother sues the manufacturers, who say they are not to blame as there is a warning on the package. Are they right?
4. A woman has a sterilisation but it is poorly done and she has a healthy child. Can she sue in negligence?

An outline answer is given at the end of the chapter.

The structure of the courts

The use of precedent is seen as:

- giving certainty to the law;
- preventing arbitrary decisions;
- maintaining equality;
- providing a rational basis for decision making.

A court is bound by precedent where the decision of a higher court is materially similar to a case being considered in a lower court. Senior judges ensure that this rule is rigidly enforced.

The courts are structured on a hierarchical system (see Figure 1.6) that allows a series of appeals in the same case.

It is essential in your study of law and nursing to look carefully at which courts the case has been heard in and inform your practice by reference to the decision in the most

Figure 1.4: First page of the Nursing and Midwifery Order 2001, with its constituent parts labelled.

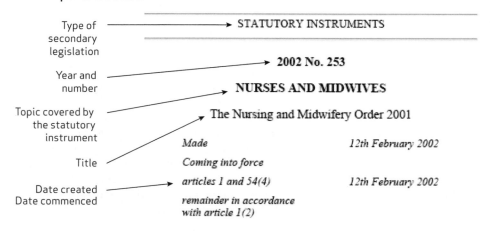

Type of secondary legislation → STATUTORY INSTRUMENTS

Year and number → 2002 No. 253

Topic covered by the statutory instrument → NURSES AND MIDWIVES

Title → The Nursing and Midwifery Order 2001

Made	*12th February 2002*
Coming into force	
Date created / Date commenced → *articles 1 and 54(4)*	*12th February 2002*
remainder in accordance with article 1(2)	

At the Court at Buckingham Palace, the 12th day of February 2002

Present,

Authority for the statutory instrument → The Queen's Most Excellent Majesty in Council

Whereas a draft of this Order in Council has been approved by a resolution of each House of Parliament in accordance with section 62(9) of the Health Act 1999;

Now, therefore, Her Majesty, in exercise of the powers conferred upon Her by sections 60 and 62(4) of that Act, and of all other powers enabling Her in that behalf, is pleased, by and with the advice of Her Privy Council, to order, and it is hereby ordered, as follows:

Part → PART I

GENERAL

Citation and commencement

Article number → 1. - (1) This Order may be cited as the Nursing and Midwifery Order 2001.

(2) This article and article 54(4) come into force on the day on which this Order is made and the other provisions of this Order shall come into force on such day as the Secretary of State may specify.

(3) Different days may be specified under paragraph (2) for different

Figure 1.5: Three components of governance.

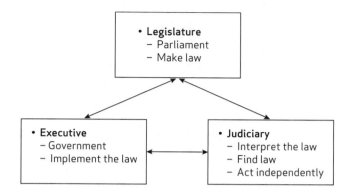

senior court. For example, in *Gillick v West Norfolk and Wisbech AHA* [1986], the case began in the High Court, which decided that advice to doctors, that girls under the age of 16 could be given contraceptive advice and treatment without parental consent, was lawful if the girl was sufficiently mature and intelligent to make the decision herself. The Court of Appeal overruled the decision of the High Court and declared the advice unlawful. In the House of Lords the decision of the Court of Appeal was reversed and the advice was declared lawful.

As the most senior court, the House of Lords hears only some 70 cases each year. They take the time to set out a wide range of guidance in their opinions that will bind future cases. Opinions in cases from the House of Lords can be reliably used to inform your practice as a nurse.

To assist with the application of the system of precedent, significant decisions of judges in cases are set out in law reports, which lawyers and those studying the law can use to inform their practice. There is a large number of commercial law reports available and some cases are even reported in the broadsheet newspapers. Case reports contain a lot of detail about the facts and law of a case. Many are now freely available from the websites of organisations such as the British and Irish Legal Information Institute (www.bailii.org) and they are an excellent source of primary law. Your university law library will have a wide range of law reports with cases relevant to nursing and healthcare, many of which will be mentioned in this book. Figure 1.7 shows the layout of a typical law report.

Case law is a particularly relevant source of law in healthcare as the sensitive nature of the disputes inevitably gives rise to decisions that have an impact on how you conduct your nursing practice.

Figure 1.6: The structure of the courts.

The House of Lords
The most senior domestic court
12 Lords of Appeal in Ordinary sit in benches of five judges
More commonly known as Law Lords
Hear Appeals from the Court of Appeal and in exceptional circumstances the High Court

Court of Appeal

32 Lord Justices of Appeal

Criminal Division
Hears appeals from the Crown Court

Civil Division
Hears appeals from the High Court, tribunals and certain cases from county courts

The High Court

92 Justices or Puisne Judges

Queen's Bench Division
Contract and tort
Administrative Court
Supervises the legality of decisions of inferior courts, tribunals, local authorities, Ministers of the Crown, and other public bodies and officials

Family Division
Divisional Court
Hears appeals from the magistrates' courts

Chancery Division
Divisional Court
Hears appeals from the county courts on bankruptcy and land law

Crown Court
Trials of indictable offences, appeals from magistrates' courts, cases for sentence

County Courts
Majority of civil litigation subject to nature of the claim

Magistrates' Courts
Trials of summary offences, committals to the Crown Court, family proceedings courts and youth courts

Tribunals
Hear appeals from decisions on: immigration, social security, child support, pensions, tax and land

Figure 1.7: Annotated law report.

Law report citation

[1994] 1 All ER 819

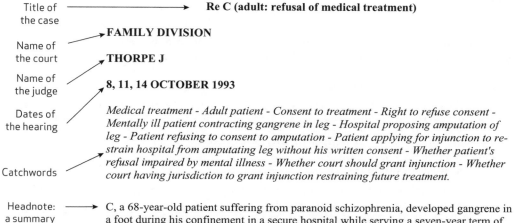

Title of the case ⟶ **Re C (adult: refusal of medical treatment)**

Name of the court ⟶ **FAMILY DIVISION**

Name of the judge ⟶ **THORPE J**

Dates of the hearing ⟶ **8, 11, 14 OCTOBER 1993**

Catchwords ⟶ *Medical treatment - Adult patient - Consent to treatment - Right to refuse consent - Mentally ill patient contracting gangrene in leg - Hospital proposing amputation of leg - Patient refusing to consent to amputation - Patient applying for injunction to restrain hospital from amputating leg without his written consent - Whether patient's refusal impaired by mental illness - Whether court should grant injunction - Whether court having jurisdiction to grant injunction restraining future treatment.*

Headnote: a summary of the facts and the law in the case ⟶ C, a 68-year-old patient suffering from paranoid schizophrenia, developed gangrene in a foot during his confinement in a secure hospital while serving a seven-year term of imprisonment. He was removed to a general hospital, where the consultant surgeon diagnosed that he was likely to die imminently if the leg was not amputated below the knee. The prognosis was that he had a 15% chance of survival without amputation. C refused to consider amputation. The hospital authorities considered whether the operation could be performed without C's consent and made arrangements for a solicitor to see him concerning his competence to give a reasoned decision. In the meantime, treatment with antibiotics and conservative surgery averted the immediate threat of imminent death but the hospital refused to give an undertaking to the solicitor that in recognition of his repeated refusals it would not amputate in any future circumstances. There was a possibility that C would develop gangrene again. An application was made on C's behalf to the court for an injunction restraining the hospital from carrying out an amputation without his express written consent. On behalf of the hospital it was contended that C's capacity to give a definitive decision had been impaired by his mental illness and that he had failed to appreciate the risk of death if the operation was not performed.

Decision of the court ⟶ **Held** - The High Court, exercising its inherent jurisdiction, could direct by way of an injunction or declaration that an individual was capable of refusing or consenting to medical treatment, including future medical treatment. However, in determining whether that person had sufficient capacity to refuse treatment, the question to be decided was whether it had been established that his capacity had been so reduced by his chronic mental illness that he did not sufficiently understand the nature, purpose and effects of the proffered medical treatment. That in turn depended on whether he had comprehended and retained information as to the proposed treatment, had believed it and had weighed it in the balance when making a choice. Although C's general capacity to make a decision had been impaired by schizophrenia, the evidence failed to establish that he lacked sufficient understanding of the nature, purpose and effects of the proposed treatment, but instead showed that he had understood and retained the relevant treatment information, believed it and had arrived at a clear choice. It followed that the presumption in favour of his right to self-determination had not been displaced. A declaration would be made accordingly (see p 822 *a* and p 824 *f* to p 825 *a d* to *f*, post).

Figure 1.7 (continued): Annotated law report.

Re T (Adult: Refusal of Medical Treatment) [1992] 4 All ER 649 and *Airedale NHS Trust v Bland* [1993] 1 All ER 821 applied.

Notes

For consent to medical treatment, see 30 *Halsbury's Laws* (4th edn reissue) para 39, and for cases on the subject, see 33 *Digest* (Reissue) 273-275, *2242-2246.*

Cases referred to in judgment

Airedale NHS Trust v Bland [1993] 1 All ER 821, [1993] AC 789, [1993] 2 WLR 316, HL. ←—— Law cases discussed in the judgment

T (adult: refusal of medical treatment), Re [1992] 4 All ER 649, [1993] Fam 95, [1992] 3 WLR 782, CA.

Originating summons

By an originating summons issued on 4 October 1993, C, a patient ←—— The lawyers arguing the case
confined to Broadmoor Hospital, sought an injunction retraining the defendants, Heatherwood Hospital, Ascot, from amputating his right leg in the present and future without his express written consent. The summons was heard in chambers but judgment was given by Thrope J in open court. The facts are set out in the judgment.

Richard Gordon and Craig Barlow (instructed by Scott-Moncrieff & Harbour, Brighton) for the plaintiff.

Adrian Hopkins (instructed by J Tickle & Co) for the defendants.
P A B Jackson (instructed by the Official Solicitor) as amicus curiae.

THORPE J.

This originating summons was issued on 4 October 1993 by C. It seeks under the court's inherent jurisdiction an injunction restraining Heatherwood Hospital, Ascot from amputating his right leg without his express written consent.

The plaintiff is 68 and of Jamaican origin. He came to England in 1956, his ←—— The judgement of the court in detail
passage being paid by the woman with whom he had lived since 1949. In 1961 she left him, and in 1962 he accosted her at work and after an altercation stabbed her. He was sentenced at the Old Bailey to seven years' imprisonment. While serving that sentence he was diagnosed as mentally ill and transferred from Brixton to Broadmoor. On admission he was diagnosed as suffering from chronic paranoid schizophrenia. He was treated both with drugs and ECT. Over the years he has mellowed and has been accommodated for the past six years on an open ward of the parole house. He is described as neat and tidy, becoming more sociable with staff and other patients in the past two years.

Table 1.1: The advantages of legal awareness to a student nurse

The legally aware student nurse:

- **Realises that many aspects of daily life are governed by law**
  Most aspects of life are regulated by law. Legal awareness helps you appreciate the importance of the legal framework which supports the structure of society. It also allows you to appreciate that personal and social problems may have a legal dimension.

- **Knowingly acts in accordance with certain legal principles**
  Many parts of the law are necessarily complex and difficult to understand. However, the underlying principles are quite simple. These affect everyone on a day-to-day basis and therefore an understanding of them is important. Indeed, ignorance of the law can bring very serious consequences.

- **Understands the key elements of the legal system**
  Knowledge of the law is of limited value unless you understand the various ways in which the legal system works to enforce the law. It is important to understand the role of those agencies that have powers to enforce the law and of the mechanisms by which you can seek legal help and advice.

- **Knows when and where to seek appropriate advice**
  The law is vast and constantly changing. You need to develop a sense of:
  - when the law can help or hinder;
  - what you can find out for yourself and where;
  - when you should seek expert help;
  - how to get the appropriate help or advice.

- **Understands the nature of law**
  Even though many day-to-day situations have a legal dimension, there are some problems that the law can do little about, even when in theory this should not be the case.

Ethics in nursing practice

In the healthcare context, nurses are expected to practise in a way that is accepted by law and their *Code* (NMC, 2008). However, you will also find that the law does not provide the answer to the complex dilemmas you will face as a nurse. Some situations give rise to questions about whether a nursing intervention is morally acceptable and ethically right. For example, a nurse may believe that a doctor's decision not to resuscitate a patient with a terminal and painful illness is wrong. The nurse may believe the patient's life should be sustained and is suddenly faced with a dilemma about what is right or wrong. Both the doctor's decision to withhold resuscitation and the nurse's desire to continue treatment to preserve life are lawful. Neither is proposing to act unlawfully and so the decision is one of morality.

Morals are influenced not only by the law but by our culture, religion and experience. As a nurse you will find that some clinical decisions are morally acceptable to you while others are not.

To develop an understanding of ethics and morality it is essential that these dilemmas are explored and analysed to provide clarity where there is conflict. This will help you judge whether a decision is right or wrong and inform your practice.

Moral issues and ethical approaches

Before we move on to consider what moral issues are and how they may be addressed, complete Activity 1.5.

Activity 1.5

A moral dilemma

A couple, both in their eighties, have been living in a residential home for about seven years. They have been married for 60 years and have rarely been apart from each other. The wife is totally blind and hard of hearing and also uses a wheelchair. When the husband's health starts to deteriorate they both ask the nurses to ensure that the wife is present during the last hours of his life. They both say that they would like to hold each other's hands before being separated.

One day, at about 5 a.m., the husband's health starts to deteriorate very rapidly. The nurses decide to bring his wife to his bedside and allow them to spend some precious time together. This was their expressed wish. While a nurse is trying to take the wife to her husband's room, the wheelchair breaks. The nurse has to look for another one and, by that time, the husband has already passed away. All the nurses on duty become very concerned about what to tell the wife. They know that, if the wife is told the truth, that her husband has died, she will be very upset at not being with him at the time of his death. Or they could lie to her, let her believe that her husband is still alive, let her hold her husband's hands for a while and then tell her that he has just passed away.

What would you do in this situation? Write down what you believe should be the decisions made to deal with this situation and give the reasons for whatever you decide. The aim of this exercise is to allow you to think about what you believe is right or wrong.

An outline answer is given at the end of the chapter.

Activity 1.6

Ethical principles

The examples in the brief answer at the end of the chapter are some of the principles that you are likely to have considered when addressing the moral dilemma in Activity 1.5. Look again at what you have written and tick any issues that are more or less similar to those highlighted in the suggested answer.

As this is for your own observation and experience, there is no outline answer at the end of the chapter.

The principles listed in the suggested answer on p29 are examples of ethical approaches that can be used to judge the right or wrong of a decision in a situation where there is a moral dilemma. The approaches do not provide you with an answer; rather, they help you to decide about whether a course of action is right or wrong. They enhance your ability to analyse situations and make a decision based on the moral principles underpinning nursing practice.

Morals and ethics

Now that you have some understanding about moral issues and ethical theories, it is important to have a clearer understanding of the term 'morals' and 'ethics'. Write down your understanding of the term 'moral' and the term 'ethics'.

Morals and ethics

According to Thompson et al. (2000), 'morals' and 'ethics' are terms used to refer to social customs regarding the rights and wrongs, in theory and practice, of human behaviour. 'Moral' refers to what a person believes is right or wrong based on their culture, experience, upbringing, education and religion. For example, a person may believe that the sanctity of human life should always be respected and all patients should be treated even if they refuse to give consent. Others may believe that the sanctity of human life should not be respected where it merely prolongs the suffering of the person, such as in cases of patients with terminal illness and in intractable pain. A person's morals are founded on their beliefs and values, and decisions made by that individual will be influenced by those beliefs and values. As a nurse you will have your own set of beliefs and values – your own moral background – that will influence your decisions when caring for a person.

Should we treat the patient?

A patient has been admitted to the accident and emergency department after a road traffic accident. He has sustained some severe injuries and requires a blood transfusion. He is conscious and understands the nature of his injuries and the need for a life-saving blood transfusion. However, he refuses to consent to such treatment despite being fully aware that his life is at risk. In about an hour he will lapse into unconsciousness and eventually die. His wife and two children have arrived at the hospital and they are all begging the doctor in charge of his treatment to save his life. They are obviously very distressed at the thought of possibly losing someone they all love. However, the doctor decides not to administer the blood transfusion even if this will lead to the man's death.

Write down what moral issues may arise from this scenario. Then write down what you believe should be done in this situation and why.

As this is for your own observation and experience, there is no outline answer at the end of the chapter.

You may think that it is morally wrong not to treat a patient who has refused a life-saving blood transfusion. This may well be based on the belief that the sanctity of life should be respected at all times. The decision in allowing the patient to die may be uncomfortable for you. You may want to force your views and beliefs about the sanctity of life on to the patient and doctor. You may even consider ways of forcing the patient to have the blood transfusion. You may consider his wife and children and feel that their wishes should be respected. All these are what you believe are the right things to consider and act upon. However, what you consider to be right could in itself be immoral. It could be argued that the patient has a right to refuse treatment and that his autonomy should be respected. As such, a patient must not be forced to accept treatment just because others believe it is right. Such coercion may be viewed as unprofessional, unlawful and immoral. This gives rise to a moral dilemma that needs to be considered. A moral dilemma, according to Thompson et al. (2000), is a choice between two equally unsatisfactory alternatives. For example, you may believe that a patient is capable of making a decision to refuse treatment and this should be respected (respect for autonomy). Another nurse may believe that one must always act in a way that promotes the well-being of others and decide to treat him despite his refusal to consent to that treatment.

This is where ethics and the application of ethical principles will help you to judge the right or wrong of a decision.

According to Edwards (1996), ethics may be described as the enquiry into moral situations and the language employed to describe them. Therefore, ethics involves the application of principles to a moral problem in order to help judge if an action is right or wrong.

A principle-based approach to ethical decision making

A common approach to the ethics of healthcare was developed by the American philosophers, Beauchamp and Childress (1989), and is based on four prima facie moral principles and attention to their application.

The four principles approach argues that, whatever our personal philosophy, politics, religion, moral theory or life stance, we will be able to commit ourselves to these four prima facie moral principles. The four principles are considered to encompass most of the moral issues that arise in healthcare.

'Prima facie' means that the principle is binding unless it conflicts with another moral principle – if it does you will have to choose between them. The four principles approach does not provide a method for choosing the right answer to a moral dilemma, but it will provide a common set of moral commitments, a common moral language and a common set of moral issues (Gillon, 1994).

The four moral principles (Beauchamp and Childress, 1989) are:

- **respect for autonomy** – respect for the right of an individual to decide for him- or herself;
- **non-maleficence** – obligation not to harm others;
- **beneficence** – acting in ways that promote the well-being of others;
- **justice** – obligation to treat others fairly.

Autonomy

The first principle, respect for autonomy, requires respect for the choice made by an individual. In a healthcare context, this means that a patient has a right to decide whether or not to undergo any healthcare intervention, even if the refusal will lead to harm or death. The term 'autonomy' is derived from the Greek meaning 'self-governing'. It refers to the capacity of an individual to make an informed and uncoerced decision about his or her future. Autonomy is about self-rule with no control, undue influence or interference from others, and it respects an individual's choice based on his or her own values and beliefs.

Gillon (1994) referred to three concepts of autonomy:

- **autonomy of thought** involves deciding for oneself using all available information and weighing this information;
- **autonomy of will** involves the intention to do something as a result of a decision;
- **autonomy of action** involves doing something based on one's decision, such as refusing to consent to treatment.

Beneficence and non-maleficence

Gillon (1994) argues that, whenever a health professional tries to help others, they inevitably risk harming them. Nurses must therefore consider the principles of beneficence and non-maleficence together with the aim of ensuring benefit to the patient rather than harm.

The NMC's *Code* (2008) underpins a moral and professional obligation to provide overall benefit to patients with minimal harm – that is, beneficence with non-maleficence. To achieve this, nurses are committed to a wide range of obligations. Nurses must ensure that they are able to deliver competent safe care and thus need rigorous and effective education and training both before and during their professional careers. They must also ensure that nursing care is of benefit to the patient. In doing this, nurses must respect the patient's autonomy. What constitutes benefit for one patient may be harm for another. For example, a mastectomy may constitute an overall benefit for one woman with breast cancer, while for another the destruction of part of her femininity may be so harmful that it cannot be outweighed by the prospect of extended life expectancy.

Justice

The fourth principle is justice – that is, an obligation to treat others fairly. Justice includes the principles of fairness, equity and an entitlement to what is deserved. Gillon (1994) suggests that the principle can be divided into three categories:

- **distributive justice** – fair distribution of scarce resources;
- **rights-based justice** – respect for people's rights;
- **legal justice** – respect for morally acceptable laws.

Equality is at the heart of justice; it is important to treat equals equally and to treat unequals unequally in proportion to the inequalities. In the context of the allocation of resources, conflicts exist between moral concerns such as:

- providing sufficient healthcare to meet the needs of all who need it;
- when this is impossible, distributing healthcare resources in proportion to the need for healthcare;
- allowing nurses to give priority to the needs of their patients;
- providing equal access to healthcare;
- allowing people as much choice as possible in selecting their healthcare;
- maximising the benefit produced by the available resources;
- respecting the autonomy of those who provide resources by limiting the cost to taxpayers.

All these criteria for allocating healthcare resources can be morally justified but not all can be fully met simultaneously.

Rights-based justice requires respect for patients' rights. Nurses have no special privilege as health workers to create rights for patients or decide which rights should apply. For example, a nurse's disapproval of a patient's lifestyle will not provide a morally defensible justification for refusing to care for a person with AIDS.

The principle of justice also requires nurses to obey morally acceptable laws. Even though you may disapprove of the law, you are morally obliged to obey it.

Applying the four principles

Activity 1.9

An expectant mother refuses to have an injection

MB, a patient, is 40 weeks pregnant and the baby is in a breech position. She is told that a vaginal delivery would pose serious risks to the child and that a caesarean section will improve the child's chances of survival. She has consented on more than one occasion to the operation but has subsequently withdrawn her consent on each occasion due to her irrational fear of needles. The patient is now in labour. She continues to refuse consent for the injection.

In a group apply the four principles to this situation and consider if the caesarean should proceed despite MB's objections.

As the answer depends on your observations, there is no outline answer at the end of the chapter.

Respect for autonomy

The principle of respect for autonomy entails taking into account and giving consideration to the patient's views on treatment. Autonomy is not an all or nothing concept. MB may not be fully autonomous and so not legally competent to refuse treatment, but this does not mean that ethically her views should not be considered and respected as far as possible. She has expressed her wishes clearly; she does not want a needle inserted for the anaesthetic. An autonomous decision does not have to be the correct decision, otherwise individual needs and values would not be respected. However, an autonomous decision is one that is informed: has MB been given information about the consequences of refusing treatment in a manner that she can understand? Has she been supported to weigh values and beliefs against the consequences of having or refusing treatment?

Beneficence

Nurses must act to benefit their patients. This principle may clash with the principle of autonomy when the patient makes a decision that you do not think will benefit the patient – that is, it is not in her best interests. Here we should consider both the long-term and short-term effects of overriding MB's views. In the short term, MB will be frightened to have a needle inserted in her arm and to be in hospital – this may lead her to distrust healthcare professionals in the future and to be reluctant to seek medical help. In the long term, there will be a benefit to MB in having her autonomy overridden on this occasion. Without treatment she will die along with her unborn child.

The benefits of acting in her best interests would need to be weighed against the dis-benefits of failing to respect MB's autonomy. From a legal point of view, the wishes of a competent patient cannot be overridden in their best interests.

Non-maleficence

Non-maleficence means doing no harm to the patient. MB would be harmed by forcibly restraining her in order to insert the needle for anaesthesia, but if she is not treated immediately she will die along with her child.

Which course of action would result in the greatest harm? The assessment relies on assumptions: how successful is the operation likely to be; and how likely will MB be willing and able to care for her child?

Justice

It would be relevant to consider cost-effectiveness of the treatment options for MB, and the impact the decision about her treatment has on her child. However, if she is a competent adult who refuses treatment despite acknowledging the risk to her life and that of her child, you are morally and legally obliged to respect her rights and obey the law. Where there is a conflict between a mother and unborn child, the law resolves it in favour of the mother. You would have to obey the law even though you may believe that an unborn child should have a right to be born alive.

The principle-based approach concerns autonomy, non-maleficence, beneficence and justice. Using these principles may not necessarily provide you with answers in all situations. Instead, the principles will inform your practice so that you are able to make decisions that are morally justified, professionally recognised and lawful. In the face of any conflict, it is important to remember that you must practise within legal boundaries and professional regulations.

CHAPTER SUMMARY

- A thorough and critical appreciation of the legal, ethical and professional issues affecting nursing practice is essential if you are to develop the professional awareness necessary to become a registered nurse.
- Positive rules impose a legal obligation to do or refrain from doing something. If a positive rule is breached a sanction may be imposed for breaking the law.
- Normative rules set out what a person should do.
- Healthcare sees a drawing together of normative and positive rules.
- Law is defined as a rule of human conduct imposed upon, and enforced among, the members of a given state.
- The UK is a parliamentary democracy and the laws of the country are created and amended through the Queen in Parliament.
- Once an Act has completed its parliamentary stages and becomes law, the authoritative and compelling interpretation of that statute is for judges and no one else.
- An Act of Parliament is our supreme source of law.
- To assist with the application of the system of precedent significant decisions of judges in cases are set out in law reports.
- Many situations in healthcare practice may give rise to questions about whether such practice is morally acceptable and ethically right.
- 'Moral' refers to what we believe is right or wrong and this is based on our culture, experience, upbringing, education and religion.
- 'Ethics' refers to the application of certain principles or theories to a moral problem in order to judge if an action is right or wrong.

- The application of certain ethical principles to a moral problem will enable you to judge if an action is right or wrong.
- The application of the principles will depend on their relevance to the moral conflicts being judged.

Activities: brief outline answers

1.4 Precedent in action (page 15)

1. The woman in the first case cannot sue in negligence as she has not suffered a personal injury. She discovered the wasp before drinking the lager.
2. Although the facts in this case seems very different, the case is still materially similar to the *Donoghue v Stevenson* [1932] case. The contractor owes a duty of care to other users of the footpath. They have failed to take adequate precautions to prevent a fall. It is reasonably foreseeable that a person with a visual impairment might come along the road. Harm has been caused by the contractor breaching its duty of care and so a claim in negligence is possible.
3. The facts and rules in this example appear similar but the manufacturer is arguing that the warning absolves them of their duty of care. You might argue, however, that as the fillet fish fingers are marketed towards children the manufacturer should take greater care. Should consumers be expected to mash each finger to check for bones? This case was settled out of court with a compensation payment.
4. At first glance this again appears to be a case of carelessness, but to be actionable, as in *Donoghue v Stevenson* [1932], there must be harm to the individual. The courts consider a healthy child as an economic loss not a personal injury. Mrs Donoghue would not have been able to sue in negligence if her bottle had contained water instead of a snail. Similarly, no claim for negligence would succeed for carelessness that resulted in the birth of a healthy baby.

1.5 A moral dilemma (page 22)

You have probably considered many issues when deciding what you believe is the right decision and best course of action in this situation. For example, you may believe that the wife has a right to be told the truth — that it is wrong to tell a lie whatever the circumstances and it is your duty to tell the truth. This belief may be based on factors such as your culture, your upbringing, your experience or your religion. You may also have considered what would happen if the wife found out that she had not been told the truth. Would she report you to someone in authority? Would disciplinary action be taken against you? Would she lose confidence in you and the nursing profession?

On the other hand, you may consider that the truth will hurt deeply and she might be unhappy for some considerable time. You may believe that you have a duty not to hurt her, emotionally in this case, but to ensure her happiness and well-being. As such, you feel it to be in her best interest if she is not told the truth. At least she will be happy and will have fond memories of being with her husband when he died.

Many different issues have emerged from this activity. You have had to judge what you believe is right and in doing so you have applied some key ethical principles to this moral conundrum. It is likely that you have at least considered the principles of:

- **rights** – the right of the wife to be told the truth;
- **duty** – your duty not to lie to the wife;
- **veracity** – telling the truth about what has happened;
- **consequence** – the consequence of lying to the patient;
- **beneficence** – doing good to the wife;
- **non-maleficence** – doing no harm to the wife.

Knowledge review

Now that you've worked through the chapter, how would you rate your knowledge of the following topics?

	Good	Adequate	Poor
1. The primary and secondary sources of legal material.			
2. The role of statutes in law.			
3. The role of precedent in common law.			
4. The terms 'morals' and 'ethics'.			
5. The principle-based approach to healthcare ethics.			
6. How the principle-based approach can be used when considering a moral problem relating to practice.			

Where you are not confident in your knowledge of a topic, what will you do next?

Further reading

Holland, J and Webb, J (2006) *Learning Legal Rules: A student's guide to legal method and reasoning*. London: Blackstone Press.

Journal of Medical Ethics: Journal of the Institute of Medical Ethics, BMJ Publishing.

Kennedy, I and Grubb, A (2000) *Medical Law: Text and materials*, 3rd edn. London: LexisNexis.

International Council of Nurses (ICN) (2006) *The ICN Code of Ethics for Nurses*. Geneva: ICN.

Nursing Ethics: An International Journal for Health Care Professionals, Sage Publications.

Useful websites

http://online.sagepub.com   Online subscription to *Nursing Ethics: An International Journal for Health Care Professionals.*

www.bailii.org British and Irish Legal Information Institute.

www.icn.ch/icncode International Council for Nurses.

www.nmc-uk.org Nursing and Midwifery Council.

www.rcn.org.uk Royal College of Nursing.

Chapter 2

Accountability

NMC Standards of Proficiency

This chapter will address the following NMC *Standards of Proficiency* and *Outcomes to be achieved for entry to the branch programme.*

Manage oneself, one's practice, and that of others, in accordance with The NMC Code of Professional Conduct: Standards for conduct, performance and ethics, recognising one's own abilities and limitations.

Outcomes to be achieved for entry to the branch programme:
Discuss in an informed manner the implications of professional regulation for nursing practice:

- demonstrate a basic knowledge of professional regulation and self-regulation.

Demonstrate an awareness of The NMC Code of Professional Conduct: Standards for conduct, performance and ethics:

- commit to the principle that the primary purpose of the registered nurse is to protect and serve society.

Chapter aims

By the end of this chapter you will be able to:

- define the terms 'accountability' and 'responsibility';
- state the four spheres of accountability in nursing practice;
- outline the conduct required to avoid liability in each of the four spheres of accountability in nursing practice;
- determine whether accountability can be exercised;
- evaluate the role of accountability in nursing.

Introduction

Accountability is a word that is familiar to nurses, as it is a term in almost daily use in professional practice with its inclusion in many nursing texts and trust policies. It underpins the NMC's *Code* (2008). However, despite its common use, the concept of accountability is frequently misunderstood. In a study by Savage and Moore (2004), the term 'accountability' was found to be elusive and ambiguous by participants. This may be due to phrases such as transparent accountability, bottom-up accountability and structural accountability being developed by policy makers and featured in literature. Yet accountability is a fundamental concept crucial to the protection of the public and individual patients. It is essential that the term is clearly understood by nurses as it is the means by which the law imposes standards and boundaries on professional practice.

Activity 2.1

Defining accountability

- Write down your understanding of the term 'accountability'.
- In a group discuss the meaning of 'accountability' with an emphasis on nursing practice.

Now read the following for further guidance.

Defining accountability

In their seminal work on the subject, Lewis and Batey (1982) defined accountability as:

> the fulfilment of a formal obligation to disclose to reverent others the purposes, principles, procedures, relationships, results, income and expenditures for which one has authority.

An analysis of Lewis and Batey's definition reveals the fundamental nature of accountability. The 'fulfilment of a formal obligation' suggests that accountability has its basis in law. There is a formal or legal relationship between the practitioner and the 'reverent others', or higher authorities, that hold you to account. The extent of their scrutiny is illustrated by the inclusion of 'the purposes, principles, procedures, relationships, results, income and expenditures for which one has authority' in the definition. It is not just your conduct but your competence and integrity that can also be called to account.

Put more concisely, to be accountable is to be answerable for your acts and omissions. This is the approach adopted by the NMC, the nursing regulatory body. It states in its *Code*:

> You are personally accountable for your actions and omissions in your practice and must always be able to justify your decisions.

(NMC, 2008)

Accountability is therefore defined as being answerable for your personal acts or omissions to a higher authority with whom you have a legal relationship.

Activity 2.2

Accountability v responsibility

The word 'responsibility' is often used in healthcare. Write down your understanding of the word 'responsibility'. In the first instance, try to focus on the general meaning of the word. Then apply this in the context of healthcare.

Accountability or responsibility

Accountability and responsibility are words that are often used interchangeably by nurses as though they have the same meaning. Accountability means being answerable to a higher authority for your actions. Responsibility, however, means something completely different. The *Oxford English Dictionary* defines responsibility as:

> *Having control or authority over someone or something.*

As a nurse you are responsible for your practice as you decide in what way you practise and what interventions are in the best interests of your patients. However, you do not have control or authority over who holds you to account or what you are accountable for. You are required to work within the law and according to the requirements of *The Code*. You may consider that your actions are appropriate and for the good of your patients, but the authorities that hold you to account can call on you to justify your actions. It is they, not you, who will decide if you are to be held to account. They bestow the level of accountability necessary to protect the public and your patients from harm.

Scenario 2.1

Nurse gave valium to workers to cure their aches and pains

In Reid (2004), it was reported that an occupational health nurse responsible for the welfare of workers in a biscuit factory saw nothing wrong in routinely giving valium to help them through their shift and rid them of aches and pains. The registered nurse believed his actions were in the best interests of the workers. However, the drugs were issued without prescription and without authority. When his actions came to light the nurse was dismissed by his employer and removed from the nursing register by the NMC for professional misconduct.

Exercising accountability

The NMC (2004a) argued that the purpose of the code of conduct was to inform nurses of the standard of professional conduct required of them in the *exercise of their professional accountability*. While it is true that the code sets out the standard of conduct required of the professions, it is difficult to see how accountability can be exercised.

To exercise accountability would require the practitioner to have control over what they were accountable for. It suggests that nurses can pick and choose whether they wish to be accountable for this action or that patient. This cannot be the case. The sole purpose of accountability is to protect the public and offer redress to those who have been harmed by your acts or omissions. As a nurse you are answerable to a higher authority and it is they, not you, who will decide if you are to be held to account. You cannot choose what you are accountable for.

Activity 2.3

The role of accountability

Having considered the definition and nature of accountability in nursing practice, write down what role accountability fulfils in nursing. There are at least four key roles that accountability fulfils; see if you can think of more.

Now read the following for further information.

The purpose of accountability

The principle aim of holding nurses accountable for their actions is to ensure that the public and patients are not harmed by your acts and omissions, and to provide redress to those who have been harmed. To achieve that aim accountability has:

- **A protective function** – The purpose of accountability is to protect the public from the acts or omissions of nurses that might cause harm. You can be called to account for your conduct and competence if it is thought that you have fallen below the standard required of you in law.
- **A deterrent function** – The sanctions available to the authorities that hold you to account protect the public and patients by discouraging you from acting in a way that would be considered misconduct or unlawful. A registered nurse must act at all times in a manner worthy of a nurse – in work, in public and in their private lives.
- **A regulatory function** – By making you accountable to a range of higher authorities, the law regulates your behaviour. The regulatory framework makes it clear what standard of conduct and competence you are required to comply with as a registered nurse.
- **An educative function** – Nurses who are called to account and asked to justify their actions have their cases heard in public with a view to reassuring patients that only the highest standards of practice will be tolerated. This public scrutiny of a nurse's conduct allows other members of the profession to learn from the mistakes and misconduct of others.

Scenario 2.2

Failure to meet the standard required of a nurse

In NMC (2006), it was reported that a registered nurse was struck off the professional register by a Conduct and Competence Committee when she admitted failing to give medication to a patient, even though she had signed the medication administration record, and for later that day giving a patient a drink of water causing her to choke, even though she knew from the patient's care plan that all drinks had to be thickened first because of the high risk of choking.

The committee found her behaviour to be conduct unworthy of a registered nurse.

Spheres of accountability

From Lewis and Batey's (1982) definition of accountability you will see that, as a nurse, you have a formal obligation to answer for your actions to a range of higher authorities, which have a legal relationship with you that enables them to demand that you justify your actions.

If you fail to satisfy those requirements, sanctions may be applied against you. For example, during your training, the university and the NHS Trust have legal authority over you. They can hold you to account through reasonable disciplinary measures. The sanctions they can impose could lead to dismissal from your course.

Activity 2.4

Accountability to higher authorities

List the authorities that can hold you to account in your role as a nurse. To help you with this exercise, think of the authorities that offer protection to the public, including your patients.

See Figure 2.1 below for the answers.

In order to provide maximum protection to the public and patients against the misconduct of registered nurses, four areas of law are drawn together and can individually or collectively hold you to account.

Figure 2.1 depicts these four spheres of accountability and highlights the authorities that can hold you to account as a registered nurse. In each case a legal relationship exists that allows you to be called to account for your actions.

Figure 2.1: Four spheres of accountability.

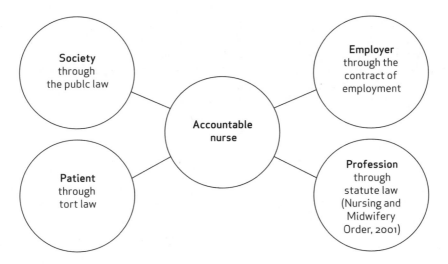

The drugs overdose

A ward sister has administered overdoses of diamorphine to hasten the death of two patients under her care. Both patients survive but suffer irreversible brain damage.

Using Figure 2.1, list the authorities that may hold the nurse to account and the possible sanctions they might bestow.

An outline answer is given at the end of the chapter.

Accountability to oneself

Very often nurses argue that they are accountable to themselves for their acts and omissions. Such an argument is characteristic of the altruistic nature of the profession. There is no question that a nurse who harms a patient through their acts or omissions will feel remorse and will reflect on their practice to prevent a recurrence. However, this cannot be regarded as a nurse truly holding themselves to account as they cannot apply sanctions and provide any redress for the person who has been wronged.

The authorities mentioned in Figure 2.1 protect the public through the powers conferred on them by the law and can apply sanctions to the nurse who fails to meet the standard imposed by the law.

The spheres of accountability are not mutually exclusive. They can individually impose sanctions on nurses who fail to meet the required legal standard. Where misconduct is particularly serious, all four spheres of accountability will impose sanctions against the nurse.

The case of Beverley Allitt

Beverley Allitt was a paediatric nurse who was convicted of killing four children and injuring five others in 1991 by injecting her victims with insulin or potassium to cause cardiac arrest (Davies, 1992).

The case was so serious that all four spheres of accountability applied and Allitt was sentenced to nine life sentences in prison; she was removed from the professional register by the nurses regulatory body; she was dismissed from her job; and the hospital where she worked paid the victims and their families compensation for the harm that Allitt had caused.

Accountability to society

As individuals working in the UK, nurses are subject to the same laws as any other member of society. There is nothing about your status as a nurse that exempts you from these laws. If you are suspected of committing a crime during the course of your practice or otherwise, you can be called to account for your actions.

Society holds you to account through the public law. Many of these laws are derived from Acts of Parliament, such as the Theft Act 1968, the Medicine Act 1968, the Offences Against the Person Act 1861 or the Mental Capacity Act 2005. These Acts are known as public general Acts and it is entirely possible to breach them in the course of your practice. Breaching a provision of a public general Act usually attracts a criminal charge, where you have to answer for your actions in a court of law.

Scenario 2.4

Accountability to society

In *R v Hinks* [2001], a care worker was convicted of theft under section 1 of the Theft Act 1968, when a jury decided that accepting gifts of sums of money from a patient in her care who had limited intelligence was a dishonest thing to do.

The patient she cared for was grateful for the way the care worker looked after him and would give Hinks gifts of money as a sign of appreciation.

However, a jury decided that accepting such gifts from a vulnerable adult was a dishonest act and convicted her of theft.

Accountability to the patient

As well as being accountable to society in general, nurses are also accountable to the individual patients under their care. The tort or civil law system allows a patient to seek redress, usually in the form of compensation, if they believe that harm has been caused to them through your negligence.

In the NHS, clinical negligence claims have a potential value of some 4 billion pounds. In 2006–7 alone some £579.3 million was paid out in connection with clinical negligence claims (NHS Litigation Authority, 2007).

Negligence

The legal expression of the ethical principle of non-maleficence is given in the law relating to negligence. A fundamental principle of healthcare ethics is that nurses should do their patients no harm. Therefore, where harm occurs as the result of a nurse's carelessness, the patient can seek redress in the form of compensation through the tort or civil law system. Negligence is a civil wrong or tort and is best defined as actionable harm. That is, a person sues for compensation because he or she has been harmed by the careless act of another person.

Duty of care

In law we are not generally required to owe a duty to be careful to just anyone. For example, there is no duty of simple rescue in England and Wales. However, in certain situations called 'duty situations', the nature of the relationship gives rise to a duty of care. The courts rely on previous cases to guide them as to when a duty of care arises. The nurse/patient relationship is recognised as giving rise to a duty situation (*Kent v Griffiths and Others* [2000]). Nurses, therefore, have a duty to take care, to be careful and not to be careless to their patients (*Bolitho v City and Hackney HA* [1998]). They owe their patients a duty of care and are accountable to the patient if they cause harm by breaching that duty.

Activity 2.6

To whom do you owe a duty of care?

- In relation to practice, list all the people to whom you believe you owe a duty of care and those to whom you believe you do not owe a duty of care.
- Discuss the reasons for owing or not owing a duty of care.

An outline answer is given at the end of the chapter.

Breach of duty

To ensure that you discharge your duty of care properly, the law imposes a standard of care on you. This professional standard is determined by reference to the case of *Bolam v Friern HMC* [1957]. Known as the *Bolam* test, it requires that skilled professionals, such as nurses, meet the standard of the ordinary skilled person exercising and professing to have that special skill or art.

If a nurse's actions are in keeping with a respected body of professional opinion, they will not have fallen below the standard required in law and there will be no liability in negligence (*Bolam v Friern HMC* [1957]).

Scenario 2.5

Patient observation

In *Hay v Grampian Health Board* [1995], a woman with a history of depressive illness, including a suicide attempt, was admitted to a psychiatric hospital for treatment. She was being kept under close observation that required that staff knew at all times where she was.

The patient was seen to be going towards the toilets and showers, and was assumed to be going to the toilets. On checking shortly afterwards, a nurse found her hanging from a shower fitment. She was resuscitated but had suffered severe brain damage.

The court found that the nurse had fallen below the standard of the ordinary nurse, as she had only assumed where the patient was. Negligence was established and damages were awarded to the patient.

Who sets the standard?

As a general rule, the courts are content to allow the profession to set the standard in accordance with the rule in *Bolam*.

However, in *Bolitho v City and Hackney HA* [1998], the House of Lords held that any expert evidence used to support this standard must stand up to logical analysis. In other words, the court has to be satisfied that the body of opinion relied on can demonstrate that the standard is evidence-based and well founded.

For example, in *Reynolds v North Tyneside HA* [2002], a nurse who followed hospital policy, which did not require a routine vaginal examination of her pregnant patient, was successfully sued for negligence when the child was born with cerebral palsy due to a prolapsed cord. Following the decision in *Bolitho* the High Court held that, while common practice was a useful guide in setting standards, it was not conclusive of the question of a breach of duty.

A nurse would not be exonerated because others too are negligent or common professional practice was slack. The court concluded that a competent nurse would have performed a vaginal examination on admission.

Inexperience

A nurse, including a student nurse, will not generally be able to argue that they are unaccountable because of a lack of experience (*Nettleship v Weston* [1971]). It is essential, therefore, that nurses realise the limits of their capabilities. Failing to refer a matter for a more senior opinion may fall below an acceptable standard of care that could result in harm to the patient (*Wilshire v Essex HA* [1988]).

The duty of care to the patient also requires nurses to keep their knowledge up to date throughout their career, although the law accepts that a period of time must be allowed for the information to come to the attention of the profession.

Scenario 2.6

The defective ampoule

In *Roe v Ministry of Health* [1954], Mr Roe was paralysed when he was injected with local anaesthetic that had been contaminated by phenol, a strong disinfectant. Ampoules of the local anaesthetic were stored in a bath of phenol, but microscopic cracks in the ampoules caused by poor transportation had allowed the disinfectant to seep in and contaminate the drug.

This was the first incident of its kind in the UK, but it had been reported in a German-language Swiss medical journal some six months earlier. Mr Roe argued that the nurses should have known about this incident. The court found that, while it was important to keep up to date, nurses could not be expected to read every journal in every language. Incidents such as this took time to come to the attention of staff and six months was too short. Mr Roe lost his case.

It can be seen that the careless omissions of a nurse are as culpable as careless acts. You can be held accountable for either in civil law.

Carelessness as a crime

Although legal proceedings for carelessness are usually instigated at civil law, it is possible to face criminal prosecution where gross negligence has occurred. As nurses owe their patients a duty of care, failing in that duty can lead to criminal prosecution if the breach of duty is grossly negligent.

In *R v Misra and Srivastava* [2004], the Court of Appeal said that a nurse would be told that grossly negligent treatment, which exposed a patient to the risk of death, and caused it, would constitute manslaughter.

Activity 2.7

Carelessness or gross negligence?

A patient from a nursing home on the Isle of Man has died of septicaemia, a form of blood poisoning, caused by infected pressure sores, some of which were the size of a fist.

- Have the care home and the nurse in charge of her care been careless in allowing pressure sores to develop?
- Do you consider that, as a result of the patient's death from septicaemia caused by these sores, the nurse in charge of her care should face a charge of gross negligence manslaughter?

An outline answer is given at the end of the chapter.

Accountability to the employer

A nurse who is employed by the NHS, or other organisation, is accountable to their employer through the contract of employment. The contract sets out the terms and conditions of employment and the standard of work expected of the employee (Rideout, 1983). Many of these terms are written in the contract, such as salary, holiday entitlement, hours of work, etc. and are known as 'express contract terms'. In addition, many conditions that regulate the relationship between employer and employee are not expressly written into the contract but are there by virtue of decided cases or employment-related legislation. These are known as 'implied contract terms' and include a warranty from the employee to the employer that they will carry out their duties with due care and diligence.

An employer is vicariously liable for the actions of its employees. That is, if an employee commits a civil wrong in the course of their employment, it is the employer who is liable to pay any compensation. Employers will wish to minimise the likelihood of that liability arising and are entitled under contract law to hold their employees to account through reasonable disciplinary procedures.

For nurses, their employer is the most likely authority to hold them to account. There are two reasons why this is the case. First, a patient with a grievance against a nurse is more likely to complain to their employer than take legal action. Second, employment law allows a lower burden of proof when deciding whether an employee is guilty of misconduct.

In criminal law, the prosecution must prove beyond reasonable doubt that a person is guilty of an offence. In civil law, the person must show on the balance of probability that a tort was committed against them. But employment law only requires that an employer hold an honest and genuine belief that the employee is guilty of misconduct based on the outcome of a reasonable investigation (*British Home Stores Ltd v Burchell* [1980]).

Scenario 2.7

An honest and genuine belief

In *This is Worcestershire* (2004), it was reported that a care assistant who was suspended then sacked over allegations of mistreating residents was fairly dismissed, according to an employment appeal tribunal.

The tribunal did not make any conclusions on the allegations of assault on 12 residents, but decided that the employer had conducted a reasonable investigation, as a result of which they held an honest and genuine belief that the care assistant had probably committed the alleged abuse.

As well as being accountable to their employer through reasonable disciplinary procedures, nurses also owe a contractual duty of care to their employers. A breach of that duty allows an action for damages for breach of contract (*Lister v Romford Ice and Cold Storage Co Ltd* [1957]). Therefore, if an employing trust pays compensation for the negligence of one of their employees, they may seek to reclaim that compensation by suing the employee for a breach of their contractual duty of care.

Professional accountability

Registered nurses are accountable to the profession through the provisions of the Nurses, Midwives and Health Visitors Act 1997, and the Nursing and Midwifery Order 2001. The NMC was established under these provisions in 2002 to protect the public by establishing standards of education, training, conduct and performance for nurses to ensure that those standards are maintained (Nursing and Midwifery Order 2001, article

3(2)). As the regulatory body for the profession, the NMC is concerned with protecting the public.

The key to the NMC's role is the professional register, where the names of those entitled to be called registered nurses are maintained. An active registration is required if a nurse intends to practise. The NMC protects the public by controlling entry on to the register through standards of training and education, and regulating a practitioner's right to remain on the register by imposing professional standards.

'Fitness to practise' is the term used by the NMC to describe a registrant's suitability to be on the register without restrictions. The NMC has the power to hold a registered practitioner to account if it is alleged that their fitness to practise is impaired. Article 22 of the Nursing and Midwifery Order 2001 states that fitness to practise may be impaired by:

- misconduct;
- lack of competence;
- a conviction or caution (including a finding of guilt by a court martial);
- physical or mental ill health;
- a finding by any other health or social care regulator or licensing body that a registrant's fitness to practise is impaired;
- a fraudulent or incorrect entry in the NMC's register.

The standards by which practitioners are judged, and which the NMC considers the public are entitled to expect, are set out in the NMC's *The Code: Standards of conduct, performance and ethics for nurses and midwives* (NMC, 2008). Practitioners who appear before the NMC's fitness to practise panels are held to account against those standards. The standard of conduct and competence expected by the NMC is that of the average practitioner, not the highest possible level of practice. This approach is similar to that adopted by the civil law when judging a skilled practitioner under the *Bolam* test to determine whether liability in negligence has arisen. The key difference between the law of negligence and professional accountability is that no action in negligence can occur without harm to the patient. A breach of the code can occur and a practitioner can be held to account even though there has been no harm to a patient.

The NMC admits that it would be impossible to compile a definitive list of the type of breaches of the code it investigates (NMC, 2004b). However, the cases regularly considered include:

- physical, sexual or verbal abuse;
- theft;
- failure to provide adequate care (for registrants who are employers and managers this can include failing to maintain an acceptable environment of care);
- failure to keep proper records;
- failure to administer medicines safely;
- deliberately concealing unsafe practice;
- committing criminal offences;
- continued lack of competence despite opportunities to improve.

As the NMC is concerned with public safety, the degree of misconduct must initially reach a level that gives rise to concern for public safety. This often means that a nurse called to account by the NMC for professional misconduct faces several different charges, which taken together give rise to a concern for public safety. The NMC expects the nurse's employer to take appropriate disciplinary action where lesser matters of misconduct, such as arriving late for work, are concerned.

Scenario 2.8

Protecting public safety

A care home manager was struck off the nursing register over a catalogue of uncaring treatment suffered by residents (Kirby, 2004). She was found guilty of seven counts of professional misconduct, including failing to take reasonable steps to maintain patients' dignity.

The Conduct and Competence Committee was told that she:

- caused up to five sets of patients' unlabelled false teeth to be kept in a box;
- failed to ensure patients were dressed in their own underwear and clothing;
- failed to ensure there were adequate stocks of incontinence pads and toilet paper;
- failed to ensure adequate care was provided for a patient with a painful sore;
- failed to ensure adequate records were kept for another patient's weight.

Investigation of complaints

Everyone has the right to make a complaint to the NMC, such as practitioners, other health professions, patients and their families, employers, managers and the public. The police are required to notify the NMC of any registered practitioner convicted of a criminal offence.

All allegations of unfitness to practise are dealt with by three NMC committees.

The Investigating Committee

Once an allegation of unfitness to practise is received by the NMC, it is initially considered by a panel of the Investigating Committee. These private hearings consider the merits of a case by reviewing the available evidence and have the power to recommend what further action needs to be taken.

The Health Committee

The Health Committee decides whether a registered nurse's fitness to practise is impaired due to their physical or mental health and, if so, what appropriate sanction is required to protect the public.

The Conduct and Competence Committee

Panels of the Conduct and Competence Committee consider allegations that have been referred to them by the Investigating or Health Committees. A panel consists of three people, with at least one member of the panel having expertise in the same area of practice and being on the same part of the register as the practitioner appearing before it.

Conduct and Competence Committee hearings are held in public, reflecting the NMC's public accountability, although parts of the case may be held in private to protect the anonymity of a victim or disclosure of confidential medical evidence. The panels are advised on points of law and issues of evidence by a legal assessor. The accused is now generally represented by a trade union officer or a lawyer. Where the practitioner chooses not to attend and is not represented, the panel has the power to proceed in their absence.

The Conduct and Competence Committee panel must decide if the case against the accused practitioner is well founded (Nursing and Midwifery Order 2001, article 29).

Currently, the panels adopt the same standard of proof as a criminal court. The facts of the case must be proven beyond reasonable doubt.

Sanctions

Where further actions need to be taken, the Nursing and Midwifery Order 2001 allows the NMC to impose a wide range of sanctions in order to protect the public from practitioners whose fitness to practise has been impaired.

As listed in article 29 of the Nursing and Midwifery Order 2001, sanctions available to the NMC where a case is well founded include:

- referring the matter to Screeners for mediation or itself undertaking mediation;
- deciding that it is not appropriate to take any further action;
- making an order directing the Registrar to strike the person concerned off the register (a 'striking-off order');
- making an order directing the Registrar to suspend the registration of the person concerned for a specified period, which shall not exceed one year (a 'suspension order');
- making an order imposing conditions with which the person concerned must comply for a specified period, which shall not exceed three years (a 'conditions of practice order');
- cautioning the person concerned for a specified period, which shall be not less than one year and not more than five years (a 'caution order').

Strengthening public confidence in the NMC

The NMC is itself regulated by the Council for Healthcare Regulatory Excellence, which oversees the disciplinary decisions of the main bodies of the healthcare professions. It has the power under section 29 of the National Health Service Reform and Health Care Professions Act 2002 to seek a judicial review of a disciplinary decision of a healthcare regulatory body where it considers that decision to be unduly lenient.

Scenario 2.9

Lenient or unduly lenient punishment

In *Council for the Regulation of Health Care Professionals v (1) The Nursing and Midwifery Council (2) Steven Truscott* [2004], the Council sought a review of the decision of the NMC to issue a caution to a paediatric nurse who downloaded adult pornographic images while on duty. The Council felt that, although Truscott was dismissed from his job, the decision of the Conduct and Competence Committee to give him a caution was unduly lenient.

The Court of Appeal held that the decision of the NMC was lenient but it was not unduly so.

It can be seen that you are accountable to the profession through the provisions of the Nursing and Midwifery Order 2001. This empowers the NMC to maintain a professional register of practitioners and to determine the standards of education and training necessary to enter the register and to establish standards for practice in order to remain on the register. The standards expected of a registered practitioner are set out in *The Code* (NMC, 2008).

The role of accountability is to hold nurses answerable for their acts or omissions to a range of higher authorities with whom there is a legal relationship that binds the nurse to their rules and regulations.

Four areas of law are drawn together to provide maximum protection to the public from the harmful acts or omissions of registered nurses. By making you accountable, the law regulates your practice and deters you from conduct that might pose a threat to the public.

It is essential that, to practise safely and avoid being held to account for your actions, you must inform your practice with the requirements of the criminal, civil and contract law, and ensure that your conduct at all times meets the provisions of the NMC's *Code*.

C H A P T E R   S U M M A R Y

- The concept of accountability is frequently misunderstood.
- To be accountable is to be answerable for your acts and omissions.
- You are personally accountable for your practice.
- You are answerable for your acts and omissions regardless of advice or directions from another professional.
- You do not have control or authority over who holds you to account or what you are accountable for.
- The purpose of accountability is to ensure that the public and patients are not harmed and to provide redress to those who have been harmed.
- To provide maximum protection to the public and patients four areas of law are drawn together and can individually or collectively hold you to account.
- A nurse will not generally be able to argue that they are unaccountable because of a lack of experience.
- The regulatory body for the profession is the Nursing and Midwifery Council (NMC), and it is concerned with protecting the public.
- Fitness to practise may be impaired by misconduct, lack of competence, a conviction or caution, physical or mental ill health, a finding by any other health or social care regulator or licensing body that a registrant's fitness to practise is impaired or a fraudulent or incorrect entry in the NMC's register.
- The NMC is itself regulated by the Council for Healthcare Regulatory Excellence, which oversees the disciplinary decisions of the main regulatory bodies of the healthcare professions.

Activities: brief outline answers

2.5 The drugs overdose (page 36)

1. Society through the public law: the nurse is likely to face a criminal charge of attempting to murder these patients. If found guilty, a term of imprisonment is the most likely punishment rather than a fine or community order.
2. The Profession through the Nursing and Midwifery Order 2001; the nurse will be asked to justify her actions by a Conduct and Competence Committee of the NMC. If guilty of professional misconduct, the most likely sanction will be a striking off order given the seriousness of the allegations.
3. The employer through the law of contract: the employer can hold the nurse accountable through reasonable disciplinary measures. An investigation of the

incident will be conducted and if her employer reasonably believes that she is guilty of misconduct, she can be dismissed by her employer for breach of contract.
4. The patient through the civil law: the patients have been left with irreversible brain damage and will argue that the Trust caring for them breached their duty of care, causing harm. They will sue for compensation in the civil courts.

2.6 To whom do you owe a duty of care? (page 37)

You owe a duty of care to:
- patients in your care;
- visitors to the ward;
- other staff with whom you are working.

If you are careless in your duties towards them, these are the people who are likely to be harmed by your negligence and so it gives rise to a duty situation.

You do not owe a duty of care to:
- patients not under your care;
- visitors to the hospital who do not come to your ward;
- other staff employed by the hospital.

If you are careless in your duties, harm to these individuals will be unlikely to happen and so a duty of care does not arise.

2.7 Carelessness or gross negligence? (page 39)

1. The nursing team have breached their duty of care towards this patient as they have been careless in failing to ensure that appropriate measures have been put in place to prevent pressure sores developing.
2. The actions of these nurses in aloowing septicaemia to devleop as the result of pressure sores is grossly negligent, so they would face a charge of manslaughter.

Knowledge review

Now that you've worked through the chapter, how would you rate your knowledge of the following topics?

	Good	Adequate	Poor
1. Definition of the terms 'accountability' and 'responsibility'.			
2. The four spheres of accountability in nursing practice.			
3. The conduct required to avoid liability in each of the four spheres of accountability in nursing practice.			
4. The role of accountability in nursing.			

Where you are not confident in your knowledge of a topic, what will you do next?

Further reading

National Health Service (NHS) Litigation Authority (2007) *Report and Accounts 2007* (HC 908). London: The Stationery Office.

Nursing and Midwifery Council (NMC) (2004) *Complaints about Unfitness to Practise: A guide for members of the public*. London: NMC.

Nursing and Midwifery Council (NMC) (2006) *Confidentiality Advice Sheet*. London: NMC.

Nursing and Midwifery Council (NMC) (2008) *The Code: Standards of conduct, performance and ethics for nurses and midwives*. London: NMC.

Useful websites

www.dh.gov.uk/publications/index   Department of Health publications.

www.nmc-uk.org   Nursing and Midwifery Council.

www.nice.org.uk   National Institute of Clinical Excellence.

Chapter 3

Equality and human rights

Chapter aims

By the end of this chapter you will be able to:

- explain what is mean by a 'right';
- describe the purpose of the Human Rights Act 1998;
- discuss how the Human Rights Act 1998 affects the delivery of healthcare;
- outline how disabled people are protected from discrimination;
- illustrate the measures enacted to outlaw discrimination on the grounds of race;
- state the role of the Equality and Human Rights Commission.

Introduction

A right is an interest recognised and protected in law. The traditional method of bestowing rights in the legal systems of the UK is to place obligations on others to act or refrain from acting in a particular way. For example, patients have a right not to be harmed when in your care. You have an obligation – a legal duty – to be careful when nursing patients. Where you fail in that duty and cause harm to the patient you will be liable in the law of negligence. In the UK, Parliament is able to create, remove and change the law and the obligations imposed by them.

Following the atrocities of the Second World War, the European Convention on Fundamental Rights and Freedoms (Council of Europe, 1950) (the Convention) was created by the Council of Europe to formalise the relationship between individuals and the government of the country in which they live. The main purpose of the convention is to limit a state's interference with the rights of the citizens, because some rights are considered so fundamental that they must be respected in every individual's case.

Activity 3.1

Defining a human right

Before reading on, write down what you understand by the term 'human rights'.

An outline answer is given at the end of the chapter.

Although the UK was an early signatory to the Convention, enforcing human rights was a difficult and protracted process as Parliament had never incorporated the Convention into domestic law. This was changed by the Human Rights Act 1998, making the main provisions of the Convention enforceable in UK law (see the box below).

Main rights incorporated into the Human Rights Act 1998

Schedule 1, part I, the Convention: Rights and Freedoms

Article 2	Right To Life
Article 3	Prohibition Of Torture
Article 4	Prohibition Of Slavery And Forced Labour
Article 5	Right To Liberty And Security
Article 6	Right To A Fair Trial
Article 7	No Punishment Without Law
Article 8	Right To Respect For Private And Family Life
Article 9	Freedom Of Thought, Conscience And Religion
Article 10	Freedom Of Expression
Article 11	Freedom Of Assembly And Association
Article 12	Right To Marry
Article 14	Prohibition Of Discrimination
Article 16	Restrictions On Political Activity Of Aliens
Article 17	Prohibition Of Abuse Of Rights
Article 18	Limitation On Use Of Restrictions On Rights

Activity 3.2

Rights and healthcare

As a group, refer to the box above containing the Rights and Freedoms contained in the Human Rights Act 1998.

- Select which rights you think should always be respected under any circumstances.
- Select which rights apply to healthcare practice and briefly give some reasons why. For example, you might select Article 5 as being relevant to healthcare because we should not deprive patients of their liberty, such as locking the main doors of a ward to prevent patients from wandering out.

An outline answer is given at the end of the chapter.

The Human Rights Act 1998 works by unlocking Convention rights, making them enforceable before UK courts and tribunals. It is unlawful for public authorities, including the NHS, to act in a way that is incompatible with these rights (Human Rights Act 1998, section 6).

The box below shows that public authorities are those that have or carry out a public function.

Main public authorities in healthcare

- Courts and tribunals
- NHS Trusts
- Private and voluntary sector contractors when undertaking public functions under contract to the NHS
- Local authorities, including Social Services
- General Practitioners (GPs), dentists, opticians and pharmacists when undertaking NHS work
- Primary Care Trusts and Local Health Boards
- Bodies that have functions of a public nature (e.g. a professional regulatory body), even if they also have private functions

How the Human Rights Act 1998 works

The laws of the UK continue to apply in the same way. The duties imposed on a nurse when caring for a patient through the laws of negligence, consent and confidentiality continue to be applied. However, where a person, such as a patient, believes that a law or the way a law is enforced breaches a fundamental right of the Convention, they can challenge that law in court. The courts supervise the decisions of public authorities when human rights are in question (*R (Mahmood) v Secretary of State for the Home Department* [2001]).

The Human Rights Act 1998 requires that all legislation is interpreted and given effect so as to comply with Convention rights, regardless of when the Act in question came into force (Human Rights Act 1998, section 3). The courts will do their best to apply this principle to avoid the need to change the law.

Scenario 3.1

Who can be a nearest relative?

In *R (on the application of SSG) v Liverpool City Council (1), Secretary of State for Health (2) and LS (Interested Party)* (2002), a woman argued that her human rights were breached by a requirement of the Mental Health Act 1983 that stipulated that in a same sex relationship the partner could not be recognised as the nearest relative unless they had lived together for five years. For heterosexual cohabitees this period was six months.

The Court held that to comply with the Human Rights Act 1998 the Mental Health Act 1983 had to be read so as to permit same sex partners the same rights as heterosexual partners. This could be done without the need to amend the law.

Where the law is in breach of a fundamental human right, then the courts will declare that it is incompatible with the Human Rights Act 1998 and leave it to Parliament to amend the offending Act (Human Rights Act 1998, section 4). This is achieved by Parliament making a remedial order to amend the legislation to bring it into line with Convention rights.

Scenario 3.2

Remedial order amending the Mental Health Act 1983

In *R (H) v Mental Health Review Tribunal for North East London Region* [2001], the Court of Appeal declared sections 72 and 73 of the Mental Health Act 1983 incompatible with the Human Rights Act 1998, as they failed to put the burden of proof for the continued detention of patients on to the health service. The Minister for Health issued a remedial order amending the sections and requiring the Mental Health Review Tribunal to discharge a patient where the hospital failed to show that the criteria for detention were met.

Obligations created by the Human Rights Act 1998

Positive obligations

Article 1 of the European Convention on Human Rights requires that steps are taken to secure fundamental rights and freedoms for citizens. This creates a positive obligation to ensure that appropriate laws and policies are in place to protect citizens and allow them to enjoy the rights and freedoms contained in the Convention.

Scenario 3.3

The law failed to protect a child from a beating

In *A v United Kingdom* [1998], an unruly nine-year-old boy was beaten by his stepfather, who was subsequently charged with assault occasioning actual bodily harm. At trial the stepfather was acquitted after the jury accepted the defence of reasonable chastisement.

Scenario 3.3 continued

The boy then took the UK Government to the European Court of Human Rights, alleging a breach of their positive obligation to protect him from inhuman and degrading treatment and punishment under article 3 of the Convention. The Court held that English law failed to protect children as it allowed the defence of reasonable chastisement and so breached article 3. The Government gave an under-taking to the court that English law would be amended to increase protection.

Negative obligations

A negative obligation requires that a state and its public authorities respect human rights in their day-to-day dealings with individuals. For example, state schools are forbidden to use corporal punishment to control unruly children.

In addition to the duties imposed by law and *The Code*, nurses also have a negative obligation not to breach the human rights of patients in their care.

Scenario 3.4

Giving treatment to a sick child against the wishes of the mother

In *Glass v United Kingdom* [2004], a severely physically and mentally disabled child (G) complained that the UK had violated his right to physical integrity under the European Convention on Human Rights 1950, article 8. On his re-admission with respiratory failure, the hospital insisted that he was dying and that diamorphine should be given to relieve his obvious distress. His mother disagreed and objected to the proposed treatment in the belief that it would harm G's chances of recovery. Diamorphine was administered but the child's condition improved and he returned home.

The court upheld the complaint that his treatment was contrary to his mother's wishes and the hospital had breached its negative obligation to respect his right to physical integrity under article 8 of the Convention.

Absolute, limited and qualified rights

Absolute rights

Not all rights within the Convention carry the same weight in law. Absolute rights such as the right to life (article 2), protection from torture, inhuman and degrading treatment and punishment (article 3), and the prohibition on slavery and enforced labour (article 4) may not be deviated from in any circumstances.

Scenario 3.5

No-lift policies and human rights

In *R (on the application of A and Others) v East Sussex County Council and Another* [2003], the High Court held that a no-lift policy, which completely banned manual handling or only allowed it where a person's life was in danger, would breach the absolute right to life (article 2) or the right to freedom from torture, inhuman and degrading treatment and punishment (article 3). The Court held that, in some circumstances, such as a fire endangering a patient's life or where a patient might be left for too long in their own excrement or might develop pressure sores if not moved, then manual handling might be the only way to protect the patient from a breach of these fundamental human rights.

Limited rights

Limited rights such as the right to liberty (article 5) have limited exceptions under explicit and finite circumstances set out in the Convention itself.

For example, if the right to liberty was absolute, then the state would not be able to imprison criminals or detain patients with mental disorders or diseases that were a danger to public health. Therefore article 5(1)(a) of the Convention allows for the lawful detention of a person after conviction by a competent court; while article 5(1)(e) provides for the lawful detention of persons for the prevention of the spreading of infectious diseases, and of persons of unsound mind.

Qualified rights

The third class of rights in the Convention are qualified rights. Qualified rights include the right to respect for private and family life (article 8), religion and belief (article 9), freedom of expression (article 10) and assembly and association (article 11).

Qualified rights have general exceptions and derogation; that is, relaxation of the legal rule is allowed where it:

- has its basis in law; and
- is done to secure a permissible aim set out in the relevant article; and
- is necessary in a democratic society to fulfil a pressing social need, pursue a legitimate aim and be proportionate to the aims being pursued.

Proportionality is a principle that requires any interference with a Convention right to be carefully designed to meet the objective in question and must not be arbitrary or unfair.

Disproportionate use of a care order

In *C and B (Children) (Care Order: Future Harm)* [2000], the Court of Appeal held that the granting of a care order in respect of two children on the grounds that their mother might cause them significant harm in the future if her mental health deteriorated was a disproportionate response to the assessed risk. The Court revoked the care orders and imposed supervision orders in their place.

Human rights and nursing practice

The right to life (article 2)

The European Court of Human Rights has stated that this right:

> ranks as one of the most fundamental provisions in the Convention... Together with Article 3 ... it ... enshrines one of the basic values of the democratic societies making up the Council of Europe.

> (NHS Trust A v M [2001])

Article 2 imposes on the state and its authorities a positive obligation to protect the right to life. The state must take appropriate steps to preserve life and this has been recognised in the healthcare context. In *Association X v United Kingdom (7154/75)* (1978), the European Commission on Human Rights stated that the concept that everyone's life shall be protected by law requires the state not only to refrain from taking life intentionally, but to take appropriate steps to safeguard life. This would suggest that article 2 covers both the intentional deprivation and careless endangering of life.

The purpose of article 2 is to emphasise the principle of the sanctity of life and, in *Pretty v DPP* [2001], a woman in the latter stages of motor neurone disease wanted a pardon for her husband if he assisted her to take her own life. The House of Lords held that article 2 gave rise to a right to life, not a right to die, and that the sanctity of life demanded by article 2 could not allow the state to sanction the intentional human intervention to end life.

The only inroad into the sanctity of human life allowed by article 2 has been the withholding of life-sustaining treatment. In *NHS Trust A v M* [2001], the High Court declared that, where the continuation of treatment was no longer in the best interests of a patient, action to discontinue that treatment would not constitute an intentional deprivation of life. The Court held that the withdrawal of treatment would not breach the positive obligation to take adequate and appropriate steps to safeguard life if that treatment was futile.

The remit of article 2 is extremely narrow. It is only engaged when there is intentional or careless human intervention to end life. Active euthanasia would be a breach of article 2. Withholding life-sustaining treatment, such as artificial hydration and nutrition, is not a breach of article 2 if continued treatment is futile or the patient chooses not to continue with such treatment.

Prohibition of torture, inhuman or degrading treatment or punishment (article 3)

Although an absolute right, article 3 contains three different thresholds, namely torture, inhuman treatment and degrading treatment. For article 3 to be engaged one of the three thresholds must be breached.

Activity 3.3

Inhuman or degrading treatment

Reflect back on your clinical practice placement and briefly highlight some instances where you believe an intervention might amount to inhuman or degrading treatment. Please do not identify the placement or the patients, but just general examples. For instance, you could write that a delay in attending to a patient who was doubly incontinent amounts to inhuman and degrading treatment.

An outline answer is given at the end of the chapter.

Torture consists of deliberate inhuman treatment, causing very serious and cruel suffering. The threshold for torture was reduced in *Selmouni v France* [1998], when the European Court of Human Rights held for the first time that a sustained beating amounted to torture not inhuman treatment. The effect of lowering the threshold for torture is to lower the threshold for inhuman and degrading treatment and, while few patients would claim to have been tortured, they will find it easier to argue that treatment was inhuman or degrading in nature.

Indeed, in *Tanko v Finland* [1994], the European Commission on Human Rights refused to exclude the possibility that a lack of proper medical care, in a case where someone is suffering from a serious illness, could amount to treatment contrary to article 3.

Inhuman treatment or punishment

Inhuman treatment or punishment is less severe than torture. It includes less serious physical assaults, inhuman detention conditions and a lack of proper medical care.

Scenario 3.7

Lack of proper treatment

In *D v United Kingdom* [1997], the European Court of Human Rights held that to deport a man in the advanced stages of AIDS would be a breach of article 3. Withdrawal of the care, support and treatment he was currently receiving in the UK would have serious consequences and would expose him to a real risk that he would die in distressing circumstances, which would amount to inhuman treatment contrary to article 3.

Degrading treatment or punishment

Treatment is degrading if it is ill-treatment that is also grossly humiliating. Treatment is capable of being degrading within the meaning of article 3, whether or not it arouses feelings of fear, anguish or inferiority in the victim. It is enough if judged by the standard of right-thinking bystanders that it would be viewed as humiliating or debasing the victim, showing a lack of respect for, or diminishing, their human dignity (*R (Burke) v GMC and Others* [2004]).

If a nurse witnessed the degrading treatment of a patient, then that would engage the patient's rights under article 3 even if the patient was too ill or incapable to be aware of the degrading treatment themselves.

The healthcare exception

A key exception to the principle of inhuman or degrading treatment applies to the provision of healthcare. In *Herczegfalvy v Austria* (1993), the European Court of Human Rights recognised that it is for medical authorities to decide on the therapeutic methods to be used, if necessary by force, to preserve the physical and mental health of patients.

A measure that is a therapeutic necessity cannot be regarded as inhuman or degrading. The Court must be satisfied that the medical necessity of the treatment is convincingly shown to exist. The interpretation of the term 'convincingly shown' by the Court of Appeal in *R (on the application of N) v M* [2002] required that:

- the decision to proceed with treatment had to be in accordance with a respected body of professional opinion as set out in *Bolam v Friern HMC* [1957]; and
- be in the best interests of the patient.

Both parts of the definition have to be complied with in order to satisfy the burden of proof that the care or treatment is medically necessary.

Therefore, inhuman or degrading treatment must attain a minimum level of severity if it is to fall within the scope of article 3. This level depends on all the circumstances of the case, such as the nature and context of the treatment, the manner and method of its execution, its duration, its physical or mental effects and, in some instances, the sex, age and state of health of the patient (*T and V v United Kingdom* (1999)).

Article 3 concerns fundamental issues of respect, dignity and humanity and can apply to healthcare.

Scenario 3.8

Refusal of psychiatric medication

In *R (PS) v G (Responsible Medical Officer)* [2003], a patient argued that her rights under article 3 were being breached because of the severe side effects of the medication she was compelled to take as a detained patient under the Mental Health Act 1983. The Court, however, ruled that the side effects did not reach the level of severity required to engage article 3 as they could be controlled with other medication.

Although article 3 has a broader remit than article 2, nevertheless it still requires a high threshold to be crossed before its provisions are engaged. Only where patients are subject to the severest forms of unnecessary distress will their rights under article 3 be engaged.

Respect for private and family life, home and correspondence (article 8)

Article 8 concerns the everyday right of individuals to respect for their private and family life, home and correspondence. However, as a qualified right article 8(2) allows scope for intrusion into this right on a variety of grounds, including the protection of health.

To be justified, any intrusion must be in accordance with the law and be proportionate to the aim being achieved.

The Convention interprets the concept of private life very broadly. In *Pretty v United Kingdom* [2002], the European Court of Human Rights held that:

> the concept of 'private life' is a broad term not susceptible to exhaustive definition. It covers the physical and psychological integrity of a person. It can sometimes embrace aspects of an individual's physical and social identity . . . Article 8 also protects a right to personal development, and the right to establish and develop relationships with other human beings and the outside world. The Court considers that the notion of personal autonomy is an important principle underlying the interpretation of its guarantees. The very essence of the Convention is respect for human dignity and human freedom.
>
> (*Pretty v United Kingdom* [2002] at [61])

As a qualified right the threshold for engagement is relatively low. Any interference with your patient or the way they live their lives needs to be justified and proportionate. For example, in *R v Bigwood* [2000], a woman was stabbed by her husband and received medical treatment and documentation of her wounds. Evidence including photographs was compiled by the police who charged the husband with wounding. The wife later retracted the complaint but the prosecution wished to proceed with the evidence they had collected. The wife argued that to do so without her permission was a breach of her right to respect for her private life. The judge agreed and the indictment was stayed.

The personal autonomy protected by article 8 means that it is for a competent patient, not the nurse or doctor, to decide what treatment they should be given in order to meet their need for dignity and avoid what the patient would find distressing. A competent patient's article 8 rights to physical and psychological integrity, to autonomy and dignity will therefore prevail over any rights or obligations located in articles 2 and 3 of the Human Rights Act 1988, schedule 1, part 1. Any positive obligations of the State under article 2 or article 3 necessarily cease at the point at which they would otherwise come into conflict with, or intrude into, the competent patient's rights of autonomy and self-determination under article 8 (*R (Burke) v GMC and Others* [2004]).

In order to show that their practice is in accordance with the law, nurses would need to demonstrate that they had followed the specific legal requirements for the care they have undertaken. For example, nurses would need to demonstrate that patients had exercised their right to self-determination by obtaining an effective consent before treatment and that they had carried out that treatment in a manner that reflected the extent of their duty of care towards the patient.

Article 8 is the most influential of the Convention articles that directly affect the provision of healthcare. It adds statutory force to the capable adult's right to self-determination – a right that can be exercised in defiance of the right to life (article 2) and right to freedom from inhuman and degrading treatment (article 3) of the Human Rights Act 1998, schedule 1, part 1.

To promote equality of rights and prevent discrimination, Parliament has enacted a range of statutes to supplement the Human Rights Act 1998. In particular, the law prohibits discrimination on the grounds of disability or race and the health service as a public body has a duty to promote equality in the provision of services. It is essential that nurses are aware of the legal and policy issues that are in place to prevent discrimination.

Disability Discrimination Act 1995

Some 20 per cent of people of working age are considered by the Government and the Disability Rights Commission to be disabled, as they have a disability or long-term health condition that has an impact on their day-to-day lives. Such people now have rights under the Disability Discrimination Act 1995 (DDA) enacted to address the discrimination that many disabled people face. Nurses have a significant role in the continuing care and support of the disabled. As part of that support it is essential that nurses are aware how the law defines a disability and what constitutes discrimination under the 1995 Act. This will enable nurses to:

- identify patients in their care who are disabled, thereby benefiting them from the provisions of the Disability Discrimination Act 1995;
- recognise an action that would be considered discriminatory under the Disability Discrimination Act 1995 and would therefore be unlawful.

The purpose of the Disability Discrimination Act 1995

The 1995 Act makes it unlawful to discriminate against disabled people in such areas as:

- employment;
- education;

- access to goods, facilities and services, including health services;
- buying or renting land or properties.

The rights of disabled people have developed incrementally. Different parts of the legislation came into effect at different times and the original 1995 Act has since been subject to a number of amendments. In April 2005, a new Disability Discrimination Act amended existing provisions by bringing a wider range of conditions under the definition of disability. It also extended the duty not to discriminate against disabled people to educational establishments, private clubs and public transport.

Definition of 'disabled'

The Disability Discrimination Act 1995, section 1, defines a person as disabled if they have a physical or mental impairment that has a substantial and long-term adverse effect on their ability to carry out normal day-to-day activities.

There are four key elements to the statutory definition of disability:

- it must be due to a physical or mental impairment;
- the impairment must have substantial adverse effects;
- the adverse effects must be long term;
- these adverse effects must affect the person's ability to carry out normal day-to-day activities.

Physical or mental impairment

The terms 'physical impairment' and 'mental impairment' are given their ordinary rather than any particular legal meaning. They can be construed by reference to what an ordinary person would regard as a physical or mental impairment. Mental impairment includes learning disabilities and mental illness. A requirement that a mental illness could only be considered if it was clinically well recognised was removed by the Disability Discrimination Act 2005, as arguments over diagnosis frequently resulted in a person being excluded from the protection offered by the Act. For example, in *Wilson v Southern Counties Fuels Ltd* (2004), a man failed in his claim that he had been dismissed due to a disability in the form of depression despite a supporting letter from his GP. The tribunal had concluded that he was not suffering from a clinically well-recognised illness and his GP did not have specialist qualifications in mental health to support his claim.

The broadening of the definition of physical and mental impairments enables many additional forms of chronic health problems to fall within the provisions of the DDA.

A disability can be due to a wide range of impairments, including:

- sensory impairments, such as those affecting sight or hearing;
- impairments with fluctuating or recurring effects, such as rheumatoid arthritis, myalgic encephalitis and chronic fatigue syndrome (CFS);
- progressive conditions, such as motor neurone disease, muscular dystrophy and dementia;
- cardiovascular diseases, including thrombosis, stroke and heart disease;
- developmental impairments, such as autistic spectrum disorders, dyslexia and dyspraxia;
- mental impairments, including mental illnesses such as depression, schizophrenia, eating disorders and some self-harming behaviours.

It is not always possible to determine whether a condition is a physical or a mental impairment. There may be adverse effects that are both physical and mental in nature, or the effects of a physical nature may stem from an underlying mental impairment, and vice versa. Some conditions, such as alcoholism and a tendency to set fires, are excluded from the Act.

It is not necessary to consider how an impairment was caused. For example, liver disease as a result of alcohol dependency would be an impairment within the meaning of the Act even though alcoholism itself is excluded.

Scenario 3.9

Depression due to alcoholism

In *Power v Panasonic UK Ltd* [2003], Mrs Power suffered from depression, which was caused by the misuse of alcohol. The employment appeal tribunal held that it was not necessary to look at causes to establish whether someone was disabled under the provisions of the Disability Discrimination Act 1995.

Particular cases or conditions

Progressive conditions

The DDA covers progressive conditions where impairments are likely to become substantial. Where a person has cancer, HIV infection or multiple sclerosis, the provisions of the Act apply from the point of diagnosis. A requirement that there had to be a noticeable effect on the person's normal day-to-day activities was removed for these conditions by the Disability Discrimination Act 2005. Similarly, a person who is certified as blind or partially sighted by a consultant ophthalmologist or registered as such with a local authority is deemed to meet the definition of disability. For all other progressive conditions the person will be treated as disabled from the moment any impairment resulting from the condition first has some effect on their ability to carry out normal day-to-day activities. The effect need not be continuous or substantial. All that needs to be shown is that there is some effect on the person's ability to carry out normal day-to-day activities (Disability Discrimination Act 1995, schedule 1, para. 8).

Past disability

The definition of 'disability' and 'disabled' includes those people who were disabled in the past but have now recovered. For example, a person who some years ago suffered a reactive depression following the loss of a loved one, but who has now recovered, is still entitled to protection from discrimination under the Disability Discrimination Act 1995, schedule 2.

Definition of 'substantial'

The requirement that an adverse effect on normal day-to-day activities should be substantial reflects the view that a disability goes beyond the normal differences in ability that may exist among people. A substantial effect is one that is more than minor or trivial.

A number of factors need to be taken into account when considering whether or not an impairment is substantial.

Time

The time taken by a person with an impairment to carry out normal day-to-day activities must be considered and compared with the time it might take to complete an activity by a person who did not have the impairment.

Cumulative effects of an impairment

An impairment may be considered substantial where its effects are on more than one activity, and build into an overall substantial adverse effect. For example, a person whose impairment causes breathing difficulties may experience minor effects on their ability to carry out activities such as getting washed and dressed, preparing a meal or travelling on public transport. Individually, these effects may be considered minor but, taken together, the cumulative result would amount to a substantial adverse effect on the person's ability to carry out normal day-to-day activities.

Effect on a person's behaviour

Account must be taken of how far a person can be expected to change their behaviour to prevent or reduce the effects of an impairment on normal day-to-day activities. For example, it would be reasonable to expect a person with chronic back pain to avoid activities such as a contact sport, but it would not be reasonable to expect them to give up their job because it involves sitting at a computer for long hours. The important consideration is what the person cannot do, or can only do with difficulty, rather than focusing on those things a person can do.

Effect of the environment

Environmental conditions may be taken into account when assessing a disability. Factors such as temperature, humidity, etc. may have an impact on the person. For example, a person who has rheumatoid arthritis may have difficulties with such day-to-day activities as walking, housework and getting washed and dressed. The effects may be particularly worse during autumn and winter months, when the weather is cold and damp, with the symptoms easing during the summer months. Although the effect on the ability to carry out normal day-to-day activities fluctuates according to the weather conditions, this person meets the definition of disability because it is likely to recur (Disability Discrimination Act 1995, schedule 1, para. 2(2)).

Treatment

Where an impairment is being treated or corrected, an assessment of disability must ignore any treatment being given to the person (Disability Discrimination Act 1995, schedule 1, para. 6(1)). That is, treatment or corrective measures are to be disregarded for the purpose of assessing a disability and this includes medical treatment and the use of a prosthesis or other aids (Disability Discrimination Act 1995, schedule 1, para. 6(2)). This applies even if the treatment results in the effects being completely under control or not at all apparent. For example, where a person with a hearing impairment wears a hearing aid, the question of whether their impairment has a substantial adverse effect is decided by what their hearing level would be without the hearing aid. Similarly, where a person with diabetes is controlled by medication or diet, the decision as to whether the effect of the disease is substantial must be made by reference to what their condition would be if they were not being treated for the condition.

The disregard of treatment or corrective measures does not apply to sight impairments corrected by spectacles or contact lenses.

Severe disfigurements

A disfigurement that consists of a tattoo or piercing is not considered a disability by the DDA. However, where an impairment consists of a severe disfigurement, such as a scar, birthmark, disease of the skin or a deformation, it will be treated as having a substantial adverse effect on the person's ability to carry out normal day-to-day activities. There will be no need for the person to demonstrate an adverse effect (Disability Discrimination Act 1995, schedule 1, para. 3).

Whether a disfigurement is severe will be a matter of the degree of the disfigurement and where the disfigurement is located. A disfiguring birthmark on the back and hidden by clothing will be considered less severe than one on a person's face.

Definition of 'long term'

The definition of disability requires the effect of the impairment to be long term. According to the Disability Discrimination Act 1995, schedule 1, para. 2, a long-term effect is one:

- that has lasted at least 12 months; or
- where the total period for which it lasts, from the time of the first onset, is likely to be at least 12 months; or
- that is likely to last for the rest of the life of the person affected.

If an impairment has had a substantial adverse effect on a person's ability to carry out normal day-to-day activities but that effect ceases, it is treated as continuing if it is likely to recur; that is, it is more likely than not that the effect will recur. This would be the case in conditions such as rheumatoid arthritis, mental illness and epilepsy.

Ability to carry out normal day-to-day activities

According to the Disability Discrimination Act 1995, schedule 1, para. 4, only an impairment that affects a person in one or more of the following ways will be considered as affecting the ability of a person to carry out normal day-to-day activities:

- mobility;
- manual dexterity;
- physical coordination;
- continence;
- ability to lift, carry or otherwise move everyday objects;
- speech, hearing or eyesight;
- memory or ability to concentrate, learn or understand;
- perception of the risk of physical danger.

Day-to-day activities are things people do on a regular or daily basis, such as shopping, reading and writing, talking, watching television, getting washed and dressed, preparing and eating food, housework, walking, travelling and taking part in social activities. They do not include work activities as work varies from person to person and cannot therefore be regarded as a normal activity. However, many types of work still involve normal day-to-day activities that would be considered when assessing whether a person has a disability, such as sitting down, standing up, walking, running, talking, writing, making a cup of tea, using everyday objects such as a keyboard or carrying everyday objects.

Scenario 3.10

Asthma attacks at work

In *Cruickshank v VAW Motorcast Ltd* [2002], a man who suffered asthma attacks at work due to fumes, but whose symptoms subsided when away from work, was held to be unfairly dismissed on the grounds of disability. The Court held that his ability to carry out normal daily activities should be considered by reference to how he was when at work, not when he was away from work.

For the purposes of the 1995 Act, fluctuating impairments should be considered in terms of their substantial and long-term effects on the ability to perform daily tasks both at work and away from work.

Discrimination

The purpose of the Disability Discrimination Act 1995 is to outlaw discrimination towards disabled people.

Activity 3.4

Discrimination

- In a group, discuss your understanding of the word 'discrimination'.
- Then discuss how a service provider, such as an NHS hospital, might discriminate against a person.

Now read below for explanations.

The word 'discrimination' comes from the Latin *discriminare*, meaning 'to distinguish between'. Discrimination is now taken to be more than distinction; it is an action based on prejudice resulting in the unfair treatment of people.

Under the Disability Discrimination Act 1995 it is unlawful to discriminate against a disabled person. Discrimination will arise when, for a reason that relates to a disabled person's disability, they are treated less favourably than others to whom that reason does not apply, and it cannot be shown that this treatment was justified (Disability Discrimination Act 1995, sections 5 and 20).

Duties as a service provider

As a service provider, according to the Disability Discrimination Act 1995, section 20, it is unlawful for the health service to discriminate against a disabled person in three key ways:

- **refusing service** – in refusing to provide, or deliberately not providing, any service that is provided to the general public;
- **standard of service** – in the standard of service provided or the manner in which it is provided;
- **terms of service** – in the terms on which a service is provided.

Refusing service

Refusing to serve or not provide a service to a disabled person for any reason related to their disability is discriminatory.

Scenario 3.11

Guide dog refused entry to café

In *Glover v Lawford* (2003), Mr Glover, who had impaired vision, was refused entry into a café with his guide dog. The café operated a policy of 'no dogs in the eating area' and this extended to guide dogs. The court held that the claimant was treated less favourably than others wishing to enter the premises without a guide dog and so had been discriminated against under the 1995 Act.

Level of service

It is unlawful to offer a disabled person a different level of service compared to other people.

Scenario 3.12

Unfair treatment of wheelchair-bound rugby fan

In Disability Rights Commission (2003), it was reported that a wheelchair user was found to be unfairly treated by a rugby union stadium, as its policy insisted that disabled people had to be accompanied by an able-bodied person. This meant they had to buy two tickets for each game, while able-bodied individuals only needed one ticket.

It is also unlawful to adopt a worse manner or use spurious reasons for doing so when serving disabled people.

Scenario 3.13

Taxi driver's bogus allergy

In Mack (2006), it was reported that a taxi driver was fined £100 and had his operator licence revoked when he refused to carry a visually impaired passenger with his guide dog, claiming he was allergic to dogs.

Terms of service

Provision of a service to a disabled person on terms that are worse than the terms offered to other people is also unlawful.

Scenario 3.14

Charging for a wheelchair at the airport

To charge customers more because they are disabled is unlawful. In *Ross v Ryanair Ltd* [2004], a disabled person was charged £18 every time he used a temporary

Scenario 3.14 continued

wheelchair at the airport. The Court of Appeal held that this was unlawful and discriminatory and awarded compensation of some £1,500.

Reasonable adjustments

Making reasonable adjustments to services, premises, employment conditions or courses of education is the key to the duty against discrimination under the Disability Discrimination Act 1995. Steps must be taken to ameliorate the person's disability so that they are treated with equality.

Each situation must be viewed on a case-by-case basis according to the requirements of the 1995 Act. The House of Lords considered the issue of reasonable adjustments under the Disability Discrimination Act 1995 in *Archibald v Fife Council* [2004]. The case concerned a street sweeper who, due to disability, could no longer do manual work and needed an office job. The council insisted that any redeployment on a higher grade must be subject to a competitive interview. Ms Archibald argued that she should be transferred straight to a suitable post as a reasonable adjustment to her working conditions.

The House of Lords held that the Disability Discrimination Act 1995 was fundamentally different from the Sex Discrimination Act 1975 and the Race Relations Act 1976. The latter two Acts require people to be treated the same regardless of race or gender. The Disability Discrimination Act 1995, however, does not regard the differences between the disabled and others as irrelevant. It requires reasonable adjustments to be made to cater for the specific needs of the disabled. It does not only permit the favourable treatment of disabled people, but demands it to the extent required to meet the duty to make reasonable adjustments.

There is no longer any justification for failing to make reasonable adjustments under the Disability Discrimination Act 1995. Dismissing a person with a disability without attempting to make reasonable adjustments is direct discrimination and can never be justified (Disability Discrimination Act 1995, section 3A(5)).

Scenario 3.15

Direct discrimination on the grounds of disability

In *Tudor v Spen Corner Veterinary Centre* (2006), an Employment Tribunal found an employer had directly discriminated against an employee, an animal nursing assistant, when they immediately dismissed her after she lost sight in both eyes. The employer had made generalised and stereotypical assumptions about visually impaired people and did not look at the circumstances of the particular case or consider what reasonable adjustments could be made to help the visually impaired person in her role.

Justifying less favourable treatment

There are instances where less favourable treatment to a disabled person could be justified, but less favourable treatment cannot be justified until the duty to provide reasonable adjustments has been complied with.

To justify less favourable treatment to a disabled person it must be shown that reasonable adjustments cannot be made on the grounds of:

- health and safety;
- inability to give an informed consent;
- inability to enter into an enforceable agreement;
- inability to provide a service to others by serving the disabled person;
- necessity to provide service on different terms in order to serve the disabled person and others;
- greater expense.

Scenario 3.16

Discrimination of a diabetic bakery worker

In *Western Daily Press* (2006), it was reported that, when a bakery worker was seen drinking a can of cola to boost her sugar levels because of diabetes, she was immediately dismissed by her employer on the grounds of disability, which they justified as necessary on the grounds of health and safety. The company settled Mrs Morrison's claim out of court, accepting that they had directly discriminated against her. They had not attempted to consider reasonable adjustments and the health and safety justification was found to be a spurious excuse.

General duty of public bodies

Disability equality duty

There is a legal duty on all public sector organisations to promote equality of opportunity for disabled people. This disability equality duty applies to the NHS and covers the full range of what public sector organisations do, including policy making and services that are delivered to the public. It requires public authorities when carrying out their functions to have due regard to the following needs.

- **To promote equality of opportunity between disabled people and other people.** For example, nurses may find that people with learning disabilities are generally poor attendees at clinics. Those responsible for delivering the clinic programme will have to ensure that the service is designed to offer the same opportunities to disabled people as to others. This could be done by working together to look at how the disability equality duty can be met. A key part of this work would involve drawing on advice from people with learning disabilities on how clinics could be made more accessible. An impact assessment will also help to identify what aspects of the clinics may disadvantage the disabled.
- **To eliminate discrimination that is unlawful under the Disability Discrimination Act 1995.** This reinforces the reasonable adjustment duties of the Act. It complements the existing anticipatory duty to make reasonable adjustments by requiring adjustments to be made in advance of disabled people attempting to use the service.
- **To eliminate disability-related harassment.** This will require health organisations to have an anti-harassment policy and ensure that staff receive training in disability equality and managing disabled patients, including those in distress.

- To promote positive attitudes towards disabled people.
- To encourage participation by disabled people in public life.
- **To take steps to take account of disabled persons' disabilities, even where that involves treating disabled persons more favourably than other persons.** For example, if a hospital trust allows cancer patients who travel regularly to hospital for treatment to be exempt from hospital car parking charges, they would be treating cancer patients more favourably than non-disabled people, but this could be justified on the grounds of ensuring that such frequent clinic attendees have fair access to services.

Public authorities must have published a Disability Equality Scheme, which must include:

- a statement of how disabled people have been involved in developing the scheme;
- an action plan that includes practical ways in which improvements will be made;
- the arrangements in place for gathering information about how the public sector organisation has performed in meeting its targets on disability equality.

Race equality duty

Discrimination on grounds of race, ethnicity, colour and national origin can have devastating consequences for the individual concerned and can lead to exclusion from full participation in society. For example, there is higher unemployment among working-age Bangladeshi and Pakistani women, who are four times as likely to be unemployed as white British women. This exclusion can in turn lead to poverty and poor health (Nazroo, 2001).

Racism can also affect the health service more directly with equally damaging results. The independent inquiry (David Bennett Inquiry, 2003) into the death of David Bennett, a Rastafarian suffering from schizophrenia, concluded that there was evidence of racism through the lengthy period Mr Bennett was suffering from mental health problems. The inquiry found that the NHS had failed to work with his family and at times treated him with intolerance. The staff were unaware of the corrosive and cumulative effect of racist abuse upon a black patient.

Staff also have the right not to be discriminated against on the grounds of race. A midwife who complained of persistent racial discrimination received £47,000 compensation, when a tribunal found that her employing Trust did not take her concerns seriously and failed to carry out an investigation (Dimond, 2006).

Scenario 3.17

Black nurse told not to treat white baby

A nurse who was moved to different wards after a mother objected to her child being treated by a black woman won her claim of racial discrimination and received £20,000 in compensation (Payne, 2004). The nurse had been subjected to racist abuse from the mother for seven years. Instead of tackling the source, her employers moved her to other wards at the hospital to prevent her coming into contact with the mother, whose child required regular treatment for cystic fibrosis.

Discrimination on the grounds of race was outlawed by the Race Relations Act 1976, which emphasised the commitment of the UK to eliminating discrimination and promoting equal opportunity. The Act empowered individuals to seek justice in cases of perceived or actual discrimination on the grounds of race.

The Race Relations Act 1976 prohibits discrimination on racial grounds. Treating someone less favourably because of race is unlawful. Racial grounds include colour, race, nationality or ethnic or national origins. It requires the complainant to point out the discriminatory act but does not require the individual to be named. The segregation of a person on racial grounds is regarded as treating him or her less favourably. For example, if a ward sister insisted that all Asian patients were nursed in a separate bay from other patients, she would be acting unlawfully and in a directly discriminatory manner.

The Race Relations Act 1976 also forbids indirect discrimination, whereby a condition or requirement disproportionately affects people from an ethnic or racial background.

Scenario 3.18

Refusing a holiday was indirect discrimination

In *JH Walker Ltd v Hussain* [1996], a factory was found to have acted in an indirectly discriminatory way when it made a general policy of forbidding holidays during the busy summer months of June, July and August. Muslim workers who made up half the workforce were refused a one-day holiday for the important festival of Eid, as it fell in that period. The Muslim employees who took the holiday received written warnings as to their conduct. The Employment Tribunal ruled that the employer had treated the applicants unfavourably within the meaning of the Race Relations Act 1976 and an award of £1,000 compensation was made to each worker affected.

The Act prohibits victimisation of a complainant by treating them less favourably because they have brought proceedings under the Act.

Institutional racism

The murder of Stephen Lawrence highlighted the institutional aspect of discrimination. An inquiry into the way the police handled the investigation into the murder concluded that the failures of the police were due to institutional racism. It defined institutional racism as:

> The collective failure of an organisation to provide an appropriate and professional service to people because of their colour, culture or ethnic origin which can be seen or detected in processes, attitudes and behaviour which amount to discrimination through unwitting prejudice, ignorance, thoughtlessness and racist stereotyping which disadvantages minority ethnic people.
>
> (Stephen Lawrence Enquiry, 1999)

The inquiry resulted in the Race Relations Amendment Act 2000, which imposed a positive obligation on public bodies, including the NHS, to promote racial equality in all areas of their work by placing due regard to the need:

- to eliminate unlawful discrimination; and
- to promote equality of opportunity and good relations between persons of different racial groups.

The duty is mandatory and must be applied to all functions that are relevant to race equality.

All health services are required to demonstrate how they will comply with their obligations under the Race Relations Amendment Act 2000 through a Race Equality Scheme. This includes the requirement to assess the impact of its policies on racial equality and demonstrate steps taken to prohibit racial discrimination and promote equal opportunities.

Ethnicity and health

Ethnic origin is important as some health problems are specific to certain communities, for example:

- **diabetes** – Type 2 diabetes (starting in adulthood) is more common in Asians, Caribbeans and Africans than in white races; deaths from diabetes are three times higher in this group;
- **coronary heart disease** – hypertension and stroke deaths for men from the Indian subcontinent are 36 per cent higher and for women 46 per cent higher than for the population of the UK overall;
- **osteoporosis** – Asian women are more susceptible to osteoporosis than the average, while Afro-Caribbean women have particularly low rates of osteoporosis.
- **mental illness** – the hospital admission rate for mental illness in the ethnic minority population is some 9 per cent higher than for the UK population as a whole.

Accessing healthcare

People from ethnic minority communities tend not to make full use of health services compared to the population as whole. According to Nazroo (2001), the reasons include:

- some people from ethnic minority groups not having English as their first language, making it difficult for them to know what services are available and communicating with health professionals where they do use services;
- cultural difficulties; for example, many Asian women do not accept a consultation with a male doctor and are reluctant to take up cervical and breast screening services;
- cultural beliefs about, and tendency to use, traditional medicines and therapies;
- cultural pressures to hide mental illness;
- the greater likelihood of people from ethnic minority groups being unemployed or on low incomes and, therefore, as a group being more susceptible to the health disadvantages related to poverty, including poorer access to healthcare.

Equality and Human Rights Commission

The Equality and Human Rights Commission (2007) has extensive legal powers and a team of lawyers who are specialists in equality law. It is equipped to take legal action on behalf of individuals, especially where these are test cases that will test the boundaries of the law and that are likely to have a wide impact. Where there are chances to create legal precedents or to clarify and improve the law, the Commission will seek to do so. Unless there is an equality dimension, the Commission is unable to assist individuals in human rights cases. However, it is able to hold formal inquiries or take judicial review proceedings to prevent breaches of the Human Rights Act 1998 and can also join in with cases taken by others to promote human rights.

C H A P T E R S U M M A R Y

- The Human Rights Act 1998 incorporates the main provisions of the European Convention on Human Rights into British law.
- The Human Rights Act 1998 requires public authorities including the NHS to comply with Convention rights.
- Convention rights give rise to positive and negative obligations.
- Convention rights may be absolute, limited or qualified.
- The right to life prohibits intentional deprivation of life, but allows the withholding of life-sustaining treatment.
- The right to freedom from torture, inhuman or degrading treatment prohibits interventions causing unnecessary distress or loss of dignity.
- The right to respect for private and family life requires respect for a patient's autonomy and dignity.
- Some 20 per cent of adults of working age are considered to have a disability.
- Disability is defined by the Disability Discrimination Act 1995 as a physical or mental impairment that has a substantial and long-term adverse effect on the ability to carry out normal day-to-day activities.
- Each part of the definition must be met for a person to be considered disabled and given protection under the Disability Discrimination Act 1995.
- Discrimination under the Disability Discrimination Act 1995 occurs when a person is treated less favourably because of their disability and that treatment cannot be justified.
- As a public body the NHS must now comply with the Disability Equality Duty, which requires a proactive approach to ensuring that services meet the needs of disabled people.
- Discrimination on the grounds of race was outlawed by the Race Relations Act 1976.
- The Race Relations Amendment Act 2000 imposes a positive obligation on public bodies, including the NHS, to promote racial equality in all areas of their work.
- The Equality and Human Rights Commission has extensive legal powers and is able to take legal action on behalf of individuals.

Activities: brief outline answers

3.1 Defining a human right (page 48)

Human rights refer to the basic rights and freedoms to which all humans are entitled. Such rights include civil, social, economic and political rights.

3.2 Rights and healthcare (page 49)

Absolute rights such as the right to life (Article 2), protection from torture, inhuman and degrading treatment and punishment (Article 3), the prohibition on slavery and enforced labour (Article 4) may not be deviated and should be respected in all circumstances.

- Article 2, the right to life: the state has an obligation not to deprive intentionally or carelessly a person of their life and this applies to healthcare.
- Article 3, the right to protection from torture, inhuman and degrading treatment and punishment: some treatment and care may be considered as inhuman or degrading such as the use of seclusion for mental health patients or depriving a patient of nutrition and hydration.
- Article 5, the right to liberty and security of person: it is sometimes necessary to detain patients due to their mental disorder or because they have a communicable disease.
- Article 8, the right to respect for a private and family life, home and correspondence: the right to respect for a private life includes respect for the dignity and autonomy of a patient and the confidentiality of their health information.
- Article 12, the right to marry and found a family: this article may give rise to issues concerning artificial conception and the right to access such treatment on the NHS.

3.3 Inhuman or degrading treatment (page 53)

The examples you give may at first appear to be inhuman or degrading but the threshold set out in law says that treatment cannot be inhuman or degrading if it is a therapeutic necessity – that is, it is in the best interests of the patient and accords with a practice accepted by a responsible body of professionals.

Look again at your list and consider if the situations you raise meet the therapeutic necessity criteria.

Knowledge review

Now that you've worked through the chapter, how would you rate your knowledge of the following topics?

	Good	Adequate	Poor
1. Rights and obligations in healthcare.			
2. The purpose of the Human Rights Act 1998.			
3. The impact of the Human Rights Act 1998 on healthcare.			
4. The law protecting disabled people from discrimination.			
5. The measures enacted to outlaw discrimination on the grounds of race.			
6. The role of the Equality and Rights Commission.			

Where you are not confident in your knowledge of a topic, what will you do next?

Further reading

Annas, G, Marks, S, Gruskin, S and Grodin, M (2004) *Perspectives on Health and Human Rights*. London: Routledge.

McHale, J and Gallagher, A (2004) *Nursing and Human Rights*. London: Butterworths.

Useful websites

www.dh.gov.uk   Department of Health.

www.equalityhumanrights.com   Equality and Human Rights Commission.

www.nhsla.com   NHS Litigation Authority.

Chapter 4

Consent to examination and treatment

Chapter aims

By the end of this chapter you will be able to:

- discuss the relationship between the ethical principle of autonomy and the law of trespass to the person;
- outline the role of consent in healthcare;
- describe the elements of a valid consent;
- define decision-making capacity;
- discuss the provisions for providing care and treatment to a person who lacks decision-making capacity.

Introduction

Nursing is very much a hands-on, interactive profession and nurses regularly need to touch their patients in order to examine them or provide care and treatment (*F v West Berkshire HA* [1990]). The right to touch an individual is limited in law and there is an initial presumption that it must not occur without permission.

The right to self-determination

The law recognises that adults have a right to determine what will be done to their bodies (*Schloendroff v Society of New York Hospitals* [1914]). Touching a person without consent is generally unlawful and will amount to a trespass to the person or, more rarely, a criminal assault. Bodily integrity is held in very high regard by the law. Unlike other civil wrongs, such as negligence, which requires harm, any unlawful touching is actionable even if done with the best of motives. As Dame Elizabeth Butler-Sloss stated in *Re MB (Caesarean Section)* [1997]:

The right to determine what shall be done with one's own body is a fundamental right in our society. The concepts inherent in this right are the bedrock upon which the principles of self-determination and individual autonomy are based. Free individual choice in matters affecting this right should, in my opinion, be accorded very high priority.

Scenario 4.1

Saving a patient's life without permission?

In *Williamson v East London and City HA* [1998], a woman returned to hospital to have a breast implant replaced. The surgeon saw her before the operation to examine her and obtain consent for the replacement of the implant. During the examination the surgeon felt lumps under the woman's armpit, but did not say anything at this time. When in theatre the surgeon decided to look more closely at the area of concern and went on to surgically remove the lumps.

The woman sued the surgeon for trespass to the person. The court held that the surgeon should have obtained consent for the removal of the lumps during the pre-operation examination. He had proceeded without permission and this was a trespass. Some £32,000 was awarded in damages.

The situation described in Scenario 4.1 highlights the high regard in which the law holds the right to self-determination by protecting individuals from violations of bodily integrity. Arguably, the surgeon had saved the woman's life, but he had done so without permission. The damages awarded reflect the seriousness of touching a patient without permission by acting in a paternalistic way and not respecting the patient's autonomy and right to decide.

The propriety of treatment

Permission to touch a patient through obtaining consent is an important defence to a claim of unlawful touching or trespass to the person. Consent, however, provides more than a defence to a claim of trespass to the person – it goes to the very heart of the propriety of treatment.

In *Airedale NHS Trust v Bland* [1993], Lord Mustill considered:

Any invasion of the body of one person by another is potentially both a crime and a tort. How is it that nurses can with immunity perform on a consenting patient an act which would be a very serious crime if done by someone else?

The answer must be that bodily invasions in the course of proper medical treatment stand completely outside the criminal law. The reason why the consent of the patient is so important is not that it furnishes a defence in itself, but because it is usually essential to the propriety of medical treatment.

Thus, if the consent is absent, and is not dispensed with in special circumstances by operation of law, the acts of the nurse lose their immunity.
(Airedale NHS Trust v Bland [1993], Lord Mustill at 797)

Lord Mustill suggests that the very rightness of an examination or treatment is underpinned by the patient's consent. Where the action of the nurse falls outside what is considered proper treatment, those acts will lose their immunity.

Scenario 4.2

Inappropriate treatment

In *R v Ghosh* [1999], a doctor was convicted of two counts of indecent assault on a female patient. The doctor had handled her breasts on one occasion, and on a later occasion had handled her breasts, and had inserted a finger into her anus and her vagina.

The court held that the doctor's behaviour lacked propriety and so his acts did not amount to proper treatment. He was sentenced to three years' imprisonment for indecent assault.

Proper treatment

The Court of Appeal gave guidance on what constitutes proper treatment when it considered an intervention that might otherwise be inhuman or degrading treatment under article 3 of the European Convention on Human Rights 1950. In *R (on the application of N) v M* [2002], the Court held that treatment that was a medical necessity could not be inhuman or degrading as long as the medical necessity was convincingly shown to exist; that is, the treatment:

- was in accordance with a standard accepted by a responsible professional opinion – known as the *Bolam* test after *Bolam v Friern HMC* [1957]; and
- was in the patient's best interests.

If either strand is not met, the medical necessity of the treatment is not satisfied and the actions of the nurse will lose their immunity.

Quality of consent

As well as requiring nurses to restrict their touching of patients to that required in the course of proper treatment, the law also demands that the quality of consent reflects the sensitive nature of an intimate procedure.

When giving consent for such a procedure patients are entitled to expect that the nurse is qualified to carry it out.

Scenario 4.3

Breast examination by a computer technician

In *R v Tabassum* [2000], a man examined the breasts of three women after they consented to participate in a survey he said he was doing in relation to breast cancer. All the women assumed the man was medically qualified in some way as he wore a white coat, but he was not. When the women discovered this they complained to the police. The man argued that he had only touched the women in the way to which they had consented and that he had no sexual motive. The Court of Appeal held that sexual motive was irrelevant. For intimate examinations patients were entitled to a person who was qualified to carry out the procedure. As Tabassum was not medically qualified in any way, the necessary quality of the consent was absent and so the consent was not valid. Tabassum was sentenced to two years' imprisonment for indecent assault.

The principle that intimate examinations and treatments must be carried out by suitably qualified people was highlighted in the case of the deputy manager of a care home who was convicted of assaulting one of her residents. In *R v Williams* [2004], the deputy manager of a care home attempted to carry out a manual evacuation of faeces on a resident in her care. Although she had ten years' experience in the care sector, she was not qualified to carry out the procedure. The resident was left screaming in pain with Williams refusing to call a doctor as it would reflect badly on the home. The deputy manager was convicted of assault and sentenced to three months in prison.

Intimate examinations and treatment, therefore, require that:

- a suitably qualified or supervised person undertakes the procedure;
- the consent of the patient is obtained before the procedure; and
- the procedure is deemed to be proper medical treatment.

Where any of those conditions are not met, the actions of the nurse lose their immunity and both criminal and civil liability might arise.

Chaperones

Further protection for the nurse and patient against allegations of wrongdoing may be provided by the use of a chaperone.

Activity 4.1

The role of the chaperone

It is not uncommon for a nurse to be asked to act as a chaperone for a patient.

- Write down what you consider to be the role of the chaperone.
- Who do you think should fulfil that role in healthcare?

Now read below for further information.

The role of chaperones for intimate examinations and treatments was considered by the *Independent Investigation Into How The NHS Handled Allegations About the Conduct of Clifford Ayling* (DH, 2004), where a doctor was convicted of 12 counts of indecent assault on his female patients.

The inquiry found no common definition of the role of a chaperone. Four differing definitions were used (DH, 2004: para. 2.51):

- a chaperone provides a safeguard for a patient against humiliation, pain or distress during an examination and protects against verbal, physical, sexual or other abuse;
- a chaperone provides physical and emotional comfort and reassurance to a patient during sensitive and intimate examinations or treatment;
- an experienced chaperone will identify unusual or unacceptable behaviour on the part of the healthcare professional;
- a chaperone may also provide protection for the healthcare professional against potentially abusive patients.

It can be seen from these definitions that a chaperone's role may be passive, as a simple witness to the examination, or active, as someone who participates in the procedure by providing comfort and reassurance, and is skilled in identifying unacceptable behaviour.

The Ayling Inquiry (DH, 2004: paras 2.58–2.60) recommended that:

- each NHS Trust has a chaperoning policy and makes this explicit to patients and resources it accordingly;
- there must be accredited training for the role and an identified managerial lead with responsibility for the implementation of the policy;
- any reported breaches of the chaperoning policy must be formally investigated and treated, if deliberate, as a disciplinary matter;
- best practice demands that the chaperone policy must ensure that:
  - no family member or friend of a patient should be expected to undertake any formal chaperoning role;
  - the presence of a chaperone during a clinical examination and treatment must be the clearly expressed choice of a patient;
  - the patient must have the right to decline any chaperone offered if they so wish;
  - chaperoning should not be undertaken by other than trained staff: the use of untrained administrative staff as chaperones is not acceptable.

The inquiry recognised that, for primary care, the development of a chaperoning policy would have to take into account issues such as consultations in the patient's home, but a policy would nevertheless have to be produced that would allow a patient the right to have a suitably qualified chaperone present during an intimate examination or treatment. Nurses must be familiar with, and apply the requirements of, their Trust or practice policy on the use of chaperones for intimate examination and treatments.

Activity 4.2

Chaperone policy

- Obtain a copy of the chaperone policy for the Trust where you undertake clinical practice. Does it reflect the recommendations of the Ayling Inquiry?
- What action are you required to take if you are unhappy with the conduct of an examination?

An outline answer is given at the end of the chapter.

Elements of a valid consent

To be a valid defence to a claim of trespass, consent needs to satisfy three key elements. It must be:

- full;
- freely given; and
- reasonably informed.

Full consent

When obtaining consent, you must ensure that the patient agrees to all the treatment you intend to carry out. Proceeding with treatment that the patient is unaware of, or has refused to agree to, will be a trespass to the person and actionable in law (*Williamson v East London and City HA* [1998]).

Nurses must, therefore, take care to explain all the treatment or touching that will occur when obtaining consent from a patient and ensure that additional treatment or touching is subject to further consent.

Scenario 4.4

Lack of full consent

In *Devi v West Midlands RHA* [1981], a Sikh woman, aged 29 with four children, was sterilised without her consent and knowledge while undergoing an abdominal operation to repair a perforation of her uterus, because doctors felt that if she became pregnant again the womb might rupture.

The court held that the surgery had been performed without a full consent. It was clear from the evidence that the woman's religious beliefs forbade sterilisation or contraception. As a result of the sterilisation she developed a serious mental health problem and lost all libido, so that her marriage was put under strain. Having regard to her religious beliefs and cultural background, the sterilisation was a real substantial loss that had been performed without consent.

Freely given consent

Consent is an expression of autonomy and must be the free choice of the individual. It cannot be obtained by undue influence. This does not mean that a nurse cannot influence a patient's decision. Indeed, part of the nurse's role is to explain the benefits of treatment to patients in order to obtain consent. Even suggesting that, by refusing to take medicine or other treatment, the patient will get the nurse rebuked is not considered to be undue influence. In law, to be undue the influence must erode the free will of the patient. It must be so forceful that the patient excludes all other considerations when making their choice, such as in situations where a threat of force or harm forces a patient to accept treatment.

Scenario 4.5

No undue influence

In *Centre for Reproductive Medicine v U* [2002], a widow appealed against a decision permitting the destruction by a reproductive centre of her late husband's sperm, which they had surgically removed and stored. Prior to the sperm being removed, he had signed a consent form in which he had agreed that the sperm could be used after his death. He later withdrew this aspect of his consent at the request of a specialist nursing sister, when it was explained that use after death caused ethical problems.

Mrs U contended that her husband had withdrawn his consent reluctantly and only because he believed that, if he did not, treatment would cease or be postponed. She argued he had been unduly influenced by the nurse.

The court found that Mr U's withdrawal of his consent to the posthumous storage and use of his sperm had not been due to undue influence. The nurse had influenced his decision by explaining the difficulty of allowing the posthumous use of sperm, but she had not unduly influenced him. Mr U had listened to the nurse, asked questions, weighed his options and arrived at a freely given decision. Without an effective consent the continued storage and later use of his sperm had been rendered unlawful.

Undue influence may also be brought to bear by family members. Nurses must be certain that the choice being made is that of the patient and is not due to the outside influence of family members. In *Re T (Adult: Refusal of Treatment)* [1992], a woman who initially consented to an operation changed her mind following a visit from her mother, a person with strong views on the use of blood, and would only proceed without blood products. When Miss T later required a blood transfusion, the court held that her refusal of treatment had been negatived by the undue influence of her mother, that her refusal of treatment was not freely given and that the transfusion could proceed.

Reasonably informed consent

The law is clear that part of a nurse's duty of care is to give advice and information to a patient, so that the patient understands the nature of the treatment proposed and can make a rational choice (*Hills v Potter* [1983]). The courts do not distinguish between advice given in a therapeutic and non-therapeutic context (*Gold v Haringey HA* [1987]).

The basis of the duty to give information is derived from two areas of law: the law of trespass and the law of negligence.

Trespass to the person

In trespass a real or effective consent requires that the nurse explains in broad terms the nature of the treatment to the patient. As long as the broad nature of the touching has been explained, no cause of action in trespass will arise. In *Potts v NWRHA* (1983), a patient successfully sued for battery when she was led to believe that she was having a routine post-natal vaccination. In fact, she was given the long-acting contraceptive Depo-provera. If a nurse gives misinformation or false information to a patient, consent will be negatived and liability in trespass will arise.

Negligence

The second type of information required to be given to a patient concerns the risks inherent in any treatment. Here the courts have been quick to point out that a failure to disclose risks does not vitiate a real consent and no action is possible in trespass (*Hills v Potter* [1983]). The proper cause of action in disclosure of risks cases falls in negligence.

Breach in the standard of care

Nurses owe a duty to their patients to take reasonable care not to cause harm. They are required to give advice to the standard of the ordinary nurse professing to have that particular skill (*Bolam v Friern HMC* [1957]). This is tested by reference to what information a reasonable body of nurses would have given in the same circumstances. However, be mindful that the court can reject a practice if it does not stand up to logical analysis (*Bolitho v City and Hackney HA* [1997]).

Activity 4.3

Knowledge of risks

- How much information do you think a patient should be given about their treatment?
- Should they be told every last detail or just what you consider important?
- Should a patient who asks questions be told more than one who asks no questions?

An outline answer is given at the end of the chapter.

Guidance on information giving in particular circumstances has been provided by the courts and nurses would do well to inform their practice by reference to this guidance which is given in the following sections.

The unquestioning patient

The issue of how much information a patient should receive about risks was considered by the House of Lords in *Sidaway v Bethlem Royal Hospital* [1985]. In this case a woman underwent surgery for persistent pain, which carried a less than 1 per cent risk of damage to the spine even if performed properly. This risk occurred and the woman suffered severe injuries. She claimed she had not been warned of the risk and would not have consented to the surgery had she been told. Their Lordships held that the surgeon had acted in accordance with an accepted body of practice at the time and there was no negligence. The degree of information to be given to a patient about risks is based on the standard of care in *Bolam*. Sufficient information must be given to enable the patient to make a choice.

There is a two-edged duty:

- to disclose material risks; and
- to withhold information where a patient would be frightened if told all risks where the likelihood of occurrence was very small.

In *Sidaway* the risk of nerve damage was less than 1 per cent and it was accepted practice not to tell the patient so as not to alarm them.

In circumstances where the treatment involves a substantial risk of grave consequences, a patient should be told of the risk, as no prudent health professional would refrain from telling the patient of that type of risk. For example, in *Goorkani v Tayside Health Board* [1991] a doctor was found negligent for failing to tell a patient of the risk of irreversible infertility at the time of prescribing chlorambucil for Behcet's disease. The risk of infertility when used over the longer term rose to 95 per cent and this transpired in Mr Goorkani's case.

Patients making general enquiries about risks

A gloss on the general *Bolam* standard of care was introduced by the House of Lords in *Sidaway*. Lord Bridge held that, when questioned by a patient about risks involved in a particular treatment, the nurse's duty must be to answer both truthfully and as fully as the question requires. While withholding information is appropriate in these circumstances, it can be seen that the courts consider lying about risks to calm a patient would be a breach of duty.

The issue of how much information a nurse should give in response to a general enquiry about risks was considered by the Court of Appeal in *Blyth v Bloomsbury HA* [1993]. Mrs Blyth sued when she suffered side effects from the contraceptive Depo-provera. She argued that, despite asking questions, she was not told about all the side effects of that drug. The Court of Appeal held that what a patient should be told in answer to a general enquiry cannot be divorced from the *Bolam* test, any more than when no such enquiry is made. In both cases the answer must depend upon:

- the circumstances;
- the nature of the enquiry;
- the nature of the information that is available;
- the reliability of the information;
- relevance and the condition of the patient.

It can be seen, therefore, that no patient is entitled to a truly full and honest answer in response to a general inquiry. The nurse only has to answer as fully and as honestly as a respected body of professionals would have answered in those circumstances.

Patients asking specific questions about risks

A different test applies to patients who ask specific questions about risks inherent in treatment. In *Chester v Afshar* [2002], the Court of Appeal held that, when responding to specific questioning from a patient about risks, the health professional is required to answer fully and truthfully regardless of the likelihood of the risk materialising. In *Chester* the risk of nerve root damage was estimated at less than 1 per cent. However, as the patient had specifically asked about such risks and had not been given adequate advice, the doctor was found to be negligent.

As such, it can be concluded that, when a specific question is asked about risks, nurses are required to follow the judgments of Lords Bridge and Keith in *Sidaway v Bethlem Royal Hospital* [1985] to the letter. Patients are entitled to full and honest answers to specific questions.

Duty to inform of mishap

Where a mishap occurs during treatment, the nurse's duty of care requires that the patient is informed of the mishap immediately it occurs. In *Gerber v Pines* (1935), a doctor was giving an injection when the needle broke in the patient due to a muscle spasm. He did not tell the patient what had happened until he arranged for it to be removed surgically a week later. The court held that, although the injection was not negligently given, there was a breach of duty by the doctor in not informing his patient immediately of the mishap.

Should a mishap occur during treatment the nurse must inform the patient immediately.

Obtaining consent

Activity 4.4

Obtaining consent

- Note down the methods you have used to obtain consent from patients when on a clinical placement.
- What is the most common form of obtaining consent used by you?

Now read below for further information.

Nurses may obtain consent in two ways. A patient may express their consent – that is, a patient makes known their willingness to be touched. Express consent can be written or oral. Written consent is usually obtained where a procedure is invasive, such as surgery, or perceived as carrying a material risk, such as an immunisation, and is often taken by means of a consent form.

A consent form provides a degree of evidential certainty to the nurse that the patient agrees to treatment. It should not be relied on too heavily, however. Lord Donaldson, in *Re T (Adult: Refusal of Treatment)* [1982], pointed out that a consent form was only as useful as the understanding of the person signing it. When obtaining consent, whether in writing or orally, it is essential that an explanation of treatment and other material facts must be recorded in the patient's file to corroborate the consent.

The second form of consent is an implied consent. This is permission implied through the actions of the patient to a request to provide treatment. An obvious example would be a patient holding out an arm and rolling up a sleeve when asked for permission to take their blood pressure.

Scenario 4.6

Implied consent

In *O'Brien v Cunard SS Co* (1891), a woman was vaccinated against smallpox on a boat bound for Boston. Told by the doctor she should be vaccinated, she held out her arm and rolled up her sleeve to accept the injection. When she later sued for trespass the court held that consent had been implied by her actions.

It can be seen from *O'Brien* that consent is implied from the action of the patient in response to a request to give treatment. It does not mean that agreeing to come to hospital or allowing a nurse into their home implies that a patient agrees to treatment. Every episode of care or treatment must be subject to a valid consent.

Scenario 4.7

Every episode of care requires a valid consent

In *Mohr v Williams* (1905), a patient agreed to a repair on a defect to their right ear. While the patient was under anaesthetic the surgeon decided to examine the left ear and, on finding the same defect, continued the operation and repaired it. The patient sued for trespass, arguing that the surgeon did not have consent for the left ear repair. The surgeon argued that, by expressly consenting to the right ear repair, the patient had implied consent for the left ear as well.

The court disagreed with the surgeon. There was no consent and it could not be implied. Every episode of care or treatment had to have its own distinct consent. The surgeon had committed a trespass to the person.

Evidential certainty

As a matter of law each form of consent, whether it be given verbally, in writing or implied, is equally effective and it does not matter which method you use. From an evidential perspective, it is clear that a written consent provides evidence that consent was obtained. Whatever method you use to obtain consent, it is essential that your contemporaneous entry in the patient's record corroborates that consent was given and that the patient was happy to proceed with treatment. As most examinations and treatments are conducted on a one-to-one basis, a contemporaneous note of the procedure is vital to rebut any allegation of wrongdoing (*McLennan v Newcastle HA* [1992]).

Withdrawing consent

Consent is a continuous process and may be withdrawn at any time. A withdrawal of consent is indistinguishable from an initial refusal to consent. Nurses must accept that, if a patient changes their mind and refuses to continue with treatment, it must cease or trespass to the person will occur.

Where the patient then decides to continue with the treatment, it is not necessary to explain the risks inherent in the procedure all over again.

Scenario 4.8

Withdrawing consent

In *Ciarlariello v Schacter* [1991], a patient underwent a cerebral angiogram before which the doctor explained the effect and risks of the procedure. During the course of a second angiogram the patient became agitated and insisted that the procedure be stopped.

Later the patient consented to the continuation of the procedure, during which she suffered a stroke and was paralysed. The patient sued, arguing that she would not have agreed to carry on if she had been reminded of the risks.

The court held that it was impracticable to apply the same stringent requirements of informing a patient of the risks of treatment, particularly a patient under sedation, once the procedure had commenced, and that the doctor had not been negligent.

The right to decide on treatment

In *Re T (Adult: Refusal of Treatment)* [1992], the Court of Appeal held that the right to decide presupposes an ability or a capacity to do so. Decision-making capacity is the key to autonomy. If a patient has capacity, their decisions are binding on you. An adult patient with decision-making capacity has the right to accept or refuse treatment even if doing so will lead to their death. This reflects the fundamental respect for autonomy in healthcare. It is not for you to judge a capable patient's decision on treatment against your values (*Re MB (Caesarean Section)* [1997]).

Scenario 4.9

Refusal of life-sustaining blood transfusion

A 22-year-old mother died just hours after giving birth to twins, because doctors were forbidden from giving her a blood transfusion as she was a Jehovah's Witness (Attewill, 2007).

Complications set in after the birth that required an immediate emergency transfusion. Although the care team explained the consequences of not having treatment, the patient refused the blood because of her religious beliefs.

As a capable adult patient she was entitled to refuse the blood and the care team were required in law to accept her decision, even though the consequences were that the patient died.

Limits to autonomy and consent

Although the law holds respect for autonomy in high regard, the right to consent is limited by both common law and statute.

A person cannot consent to an action that would lead to their death, and a nurse who killed a patient even where the patient requested it would face a charge of murder.

Scenario 4.10

Killing a patient

In *R v Cox* (1992), a consultant gave a patient a lethal injection when she reminded him that he had promised not to let her suffer.

She was cremated before the details of the incident became known and so the doctor was only convicted of attempted murder.

It is also unlawful to assist a patient to die. Although it is not illegal to take one's own life, to aid, abet, procure or counsel the suicide of another person is unlawful and punishable by up to 14 years' imprisonment (Suicide Act 1961, section 2). This law protects the vulnerable from being encouraged to take their own life by unscrupulous relatives, friends or health professionals.

Scenario 4.11

Assisted suicide

In *R v McShane* [1977], a daughter was found guilty of trying to persuade her 89-year-old mother, who was residing in a nursing home, to kill herself so that she could inherit her mother's estate. The police obtained incriminating evidence of the daughter by using a hidden camera at the nursing home that showed the daughter handing her mother drugs, hidden in a packet of sweets, and pinning a note on her mother's dress telling her not to 'bungle it'!

Decision-making capacity

Decision-making capacity is the ability to make a decision and it is the key to autonomy (*Re T (Adult: Refusal of Treatment)* [1992]). It is based on the person understanding and using information about treatment when making a decision.

Decision-making capacity can vary over time and can vary depending on the decision to be made. A patient might have the requisite capacity to make a simple decision but not the requisite capacity to make a complex decision.

Scenario 4.12

Capacity to marry and make a will

An 84-year-old man chose to marry his 24-year-old maid when he was very ill and frail. Once married, his will became void and he made a new one bequeathing his considerable estate equally between his new wife and his adult children.

When he died a short while after, his wife knew that she would inherit considerably more of his estate if he had died without making a valid will. She argued that he did not have the capacity to make a will. His children countered by saying that, if that was the case, he did not have the capacity to marry his maid.

In *In the Estate of Park* [1953], the court held that the complexity and level of understanding required when making a will was far greater than the capacity required to agree to marry someone. The court decided that the man was capable of agreeing to marry and marrying his wife, but lacked the capacity to make a new will.

Capacity is based on a test of understanding and is not a professional or status test. You cannot assume lack of capacity because of a person's age, physical appearance, condition or an aspect of their behaviour.

Patients who lack decision-making capacity

Patients aged 16 and over are assumed in law to have the ability to make decisions about their healthcare and their consent to treatment is required before it can proceed.

Where the patient lacks decision-making capacity, the Mental Capacity Act 2005 and its guiding principles ensure that their rights and interests are at the centre of the decision-making process (see the box below).

The principles of the Mental Capacity Act 2005

- A person must be assumed to have capacity unless it is established that he or she lacks capacity.
- A person is not to be treated as unable to make a decision unless all practicable steps to help him or her to do so have been taken without success.
- A person is not to be treated as unable to make a decision merely because he or she makes an unwise decision.
- An act done, or decision made, under this Act for or on behalf of a person who lacks capacity must be done, or made, in his or her best interests.
- Before the act is done, or the decision is made, regard must be had to whether the purpose for which it is needed can be as effectively achieved in a way that is less restrictive of the person's rights and freedom of action.

The Mental Capacity Act 2005 requires you to assume that a person aged 16 or older has the capacity to make decisions, even unwise decisions, for themselves. You are able to act on a patient's decision to accept or refuse treatment without the need to assess decision-making capacity. The need to assess capacity only arises where the behaviour or circumstances of the person triggers a doubt in your mind about their ability to make a decision. The principle stresses a person's right to autonomy and is further supported by requiring steps be taken to maximise decision-making capacity.

Activity 4.5

Practical steps to help a person make decisions

The law recognises that some people require support to make decisions. What practicable steps could you take to help a person make a decision about care and treatment?

Now read below for further information.

The Code of Practice of the Mental Capacity Act 2005 (Department for Constitutional Affairs, 2007) suggests that practical steps to help a person make a decision might include:

- using simple language and, where appropriate, pictures and objects rather than words;

- arranging for the person to have the information in their preferred language;
- consulting whoever knows the person well on the best methods of communication;
- choosing the best time and location where the person feels at ease;
- waiting until the person's capacity improves before requiring a decision.

Where a person is considered to lack decision-making capacity, any action or decision taken must be in their best interests (see page 83).

The final guiding principle of the Mental Capacity Act 2005 requires you to act in the least restrictive way possible. This important requirement will ensure that any interference with a person's rights and freedom to make decisions will be limited to that required to meet the immediate needs of the individual.

Assessing decision-making capacity

A person lacks capacity where an impairment or disturbance of the mind or brain affects their ability to make a particular decision. It does not matter whether the lack of capacity is permanent or temporary.

Scenario 4.13

Temporary lack of capacity

In *Re MB (Caesarean Section)* [1997], the Court of Appeal held that the panic instilled by a needle phobia drove so forcibly into the mind of the patient that she was unable to weigh the consequences of refusing treatment and was temporarily incapable.

The test for decision-making capacity is a two-stage functional test based on the decision to be made at that time rather than a general ability to make decisions; that is:

1. Is there a permanent or temporary impairment or disturbance to the functioning of patient's mind or brain?
2. If there is, how far does it affect the person's ability to make a decision?

A person will not be capable of making a decision if, due to an impairment or disturbance to the mind or brain, they are unable to:

- understand the treatment information relevant to the decision; or
- retain the information long enough to make a decision; or
- use or weigh the information as part of the process of arriving at a decision; or
- communicate that decision by any means.

Scenario 4.14

Does the patient have decision-making capacity?

In *Re C (Adult: Refusal of Treatment)* [1994], a man detained in Broadmoor special hospital and suffering from paranoid schizophrenia, with a false belief that he was a doctor, developed gangrene in his right foot. He refused consent for an amputation and took the hospital to court to ensure that no treatment would proceed without his express consent.

The judge decided that *Mr C* had decision-making capacity, because, despite his profound mental health problem, he understood the surgeon's advice about the dangers of refusing treatment. He retained that treatment advice and repeated it back to the judge. Then he showed that he had used the treatment information when weighing up his options by telling the judge that he might die without the amputation but he was prepared to trust in God.

It will generally be for the person providing treatment to determine whether a patient has decision-making capacity. Where the issue is more serious, with many people involved in the care and treatment, the person in charge, usually the senior doctor, will determine if the patient has decision-making capacity. If a dispute over capacity remains unresolved, the courts will determine decision-making capacity.

Stages of the assessment process

The trigger phase
You must assume that a patient 16 years or older has capacity to consent to care or treatment unless a concern triggers a doubt about the person's decision-making capacity.

The practical support phase
You cannot say a person lacks decision-making capacity unless you have taken practical steps to help them to make a decision.

The diagnostic threshold
Are you able to discern an impairment or disturbance to the functioning of the person's mind or brain? It does not matter if this is permanent or temporary. If you cannot determine such an impairment or disturbance, no further action can be taken under the Mental Capacity Act 2005.

The assessment phase
How far does the impairment or disturbance to the person's mind or brain affect their ability to make a decision? Where a person cannot

- understand treatment information; or
- retain treatment information; or
- use or weigh treatment information when making a decision; or
- communicate their decision in some way; then

you can reasonably conclude that they lack capacity for that particular decision.

Designated decision makers

The Mental Capacity Act 2005 has two formal powers that allow a third party to make decisions on behalf of a person who lacks decision-making capacity. These powers can give the designated decision maker the right to consent to or refuse medical treatment. Where a designated decision maker with authority is in place for a patient, their consent must be obtained before care and treatment can lawfully be given.

Personal welfare lasting power of attorney

A power allowing another to consent on behalf of a person who lacks capacity to make decisions can be created through a personal welfare lasting power of attorney. The power must be created by the person (the donor) when they are capable and can only come into force when the person lacks capacity and the power of attorney has been registered with the Office of Public Guardian.

A person can also create a lasting power of attorney that allows another to manage their property and affairs.

Court of Protection deputy

When continuing decisions need to be made on behalf of a person who lacks capacity and there is no lasting power of attorney in place, the Court of Protection may appoint a person, called a deputy, to make personal welfare decisions on behalf of the incapable patient that can include the right to consent to or refuse treatment.

The Court must be satisfied that the deputy is willing and able to fulfil the role and that appointing a deputy is a proportionate response to the needs of the patient.

Advance decisions refusing treatment

As well as having designated decision makers able to make consent to treatment decisions, a person can make an advance refusal of treatment. Where a valid applicable advance refusal is in place, the wishes of the patient must be respected and treatment withheld. Compulsory treatment for mental disorder under the Mental Health Act 1983, other than electroconvulsive therapy (ECT), can override a valid and applicable advance decision refusing healthcare.

Scenario 4.15

Advance decision refusing treatment

In *Re AK (Adult Patient) (Medical Treatment: Consent)* [2001], a man with motor neurone disease had a long-established advance decision refusing treatment that stated that, two weeks after he lost the ability to communicate, his care team were to withhold his artificial nutrition and hydration. The court confirmed that the conditions expressed by the patient when an adult with capacity had now come into effect and it was lawful to withhold the treatment.

Although advance decisions can be made orally, where they are to apply to life-sustaining treatment, the Mental Capacity Act 2005, section 25, requires that they are:

- made in writing;
- signed by the person or signed on their behalf in their presence;
- witnessed in writing in the presence of the person;
- verified by a statement made by the maker that expressly and specifically states that the advanced decision is to apply even if life is at risk.

Best interests

The Mental Capacity Act 2005 provides a checklist of factors that must be considered when determining whether care and treatment is in the best interests of a patient who lacks capacity.

This holistic approach to best interests ensures that the wishes of the patient and views of those caring for the patient are taken into account.

When determining whether care and treatment is in an incapable patient's best interests you must:

- consider all the relevant circumstances;
- consider whether the decision can wait until the person regains capacity;
- as far as reasonably practicable, permit and encourage the person to participate in their care and treatment;
- not be motivated by a desire to bring about the death of the patient;
- consider, as far as is reasonably ascertainable:
  o the person's past and present wishes and feelings (and, in particular, any relevant written statement made when they had capacity);
  o the beliefs and values that would be likely to influence their decision if they had capacity;
  o other factors that they would be likely to consider if they were able to do so;
- take into account, if it is practicable and appropriate to consult them, the views of the following, as to what would be in the person's best interests:
  o anyone named by the person as someone to be consulted on the matter in question or on matters of that kind;
  o anyone engaged in caring for the person or interested in his or her welfare;
  o any donee of a lasting power of attorney granted by the person;
  o any deputy appointed for the person by the court.

Independent Mental Capacity Advocate

Where no suitable person is available to be consulted on what would be in the best interests of the patient, there may be a duty to instruct an Independent Mental Capacity Advocate (IMCA).

The IMCA will make representations about the person's wishes, feelings and beliefs, and call the decision maker's attention to the factors relevant to their decision.

IMCAs will only be involved where the decision concerns:

- serious medical treatment; that is, treatment that involves providing, withdrawing or withholding treatment in circumstances where:
  o in a case where a single treatment is being proposed, there is a fine balance between its benefits to the patient, and the burdens and risks it is likely to entail for him or her;
  o in a case where there is a choice of treatments, a decision as to which one to use is finely balanced; or
  o what is proposed would be likely to involve serious consequences for the patient;
- a change in the person's accommodation, where it is provided by the NHS or local authority; or
- authorised detention under the deprivation of liberty safeguards.

Protection from liability

Where care and treatment for an incapable adult proceeds following an assessment of capacity and determination of best interests, the caregiver is protected from liability in the law relating to consent.

Restraint

Restraint is defined as:

> the use or threat of force where the person is resisting and any restriction of liberty of movement whether or not the person resists.

This wide definition includes even mild forms of restraint, such as holding an incapable person's hand to prevent them wandering away and holding an arm to keep it still when taking a blood sample. Restraint is permitted but only when the person using it reasonably believes it is necessary to prevent harm to the incapable person.

The restraint used must be proportionate to both the likelihood of the harm and the seriousness of the harm.

Deprivation of liberty safeguards

There may be occasions when a person who lacks decision-making capacity is deprived of their liberty in their best interests when in hospital or a care home. To ensure that the person's human rights are respected, the deprivation of liberty must be authorised through an assessment by two health and social care professionals, including mental health nurses, to ensure that:

- the adult lacks decision-making capacity due to an impairment or disturbance of the mind or brain;
- it is in their best interests to be deprived of their liberty, taking into account any objections against such a finding;
- the person is not, or would be better protected by, being subject to compulsion under the Mental Health Act 1983, such as guardianship.

Where assessment agrees that the person should be deprived of their liberty in their best interests, this can be authorised for any period up to 12 months. A representative will be appointed who can ask for the issue to be reviewed.

Court of Protection

The Court of Protection is a specialist court that hears cases and settles matters concerning people who lack capacity. The Court can also appoint deputies (see page 87) and give them powers to make ongoing decisions for capable adults.

Office of Public Guardian

The Office of Public Guardian is responsible for the supervision of deputies appointed by the Court and for supporting deputies in their role.

It also has a role in protecting people subject to the Court's powers from abuse or exploitation by:

- keeping a register of lasting powers of attorney;
- keeping a register of orders appointing deputies;
- supervising deputies appointed by the Court;
- receiving reports from attorneys;
- dealing with enquiries and complaints about deputies and attorneys.

Research with incapable adults

Research concerning people who lack capacity, other than a clinical trial for new medicines, is regulated by the Mental Capacity Act 2005, which requires those conducting a research project to:

- satisfy a research ethics committee as to why subjects who lack decision-making capacity are to be used in the study;
- speak to a relative or friend who can veto the person's participation in the research;
- remove a subject from participation in the study if, during the study, the subject shows any resistance or distress for whatever reason.

C H A P T E R   S U M M A R Y

- The moral principle of autonomy is given its legal expression in the law relating to consent.
- Consent imposes on nurses a legal obligation to respect an individual's autonomy and self-determination.
- Consent is essential to the propriety of care and treatment.
- A legally valid consent will protect the practitioner from the tort of trespass to the person and the criminal offence of assault and battery.
- A valid consent must be full, free from duress and reasonably informed.
- An adult with decision-making capacity is able to refuse treatment even if such refusal might lead to his or her death.
- Where there is doubt about the capacity of a person 16 or older to make a treatment decision, their capacity must be assessed in accordance with the guiding principles of the Mental Capacity Act 2005.
- Treatment for a person who lacks capacity can only proceed if it is in their best interests.
- Best interests must be determined in accordance with the checklist of factors set out under the Mental Capacity Act 2005.
- The Mental Capacity Act 2005 allows for designated decision makers to consent to treatment for people who lack capacity.

Activities: brief outline answers

4.2 Chaperone policy (page 76)

- The recommendations of the Ayling Inquiry, including how to respond to an improper examination, should be reflected in this policy.
- Look carefully at the policy and identify what action is to be taken if you are unhappy with the conduct of the examination. The policy should reflect the Ayling Inquiry recommendation that a chaperone can stop the examination continuing if they are unhappy with the conduct of the examination, that the policy has a clear reporting mechanism for concerns and requires that reported breaches of the chaperoning policy be formally investigated through each Trust's risk management and clinical governance arrangements.

4.3 Knowledge of risks (page 78)

The degree of information to be given to a patient about risks is based on the standard of care in *Bolam*. Sufficient information must be given to enable the patient to make a choice. There is a two-edged duty:

- to disclose material risks;
- to withhold information where a patient would be frightened if told all risks where the likelihood of occurrence was very small.

The issue of how much information a nurse should give in response to a general enquiry about risks was considered by the Court of Appeal in *Blyth v Bloomsbury HA* [1993]. The answer depends on:

- the circumstances;
- the nature of the enquiry;
- the nature of the information which is available;
- its reliability and relevance;
- the condition of the patient.

A different test applies to patients who ask specific questions about risks inherent in treatment. When a specific question is asked about risks, patients are entitled to full and honest answers.

Knowledge review

Now that you've worked through the chapter, how would you rate your knowledge of the following topics?

	Good	Adequate	Poor
1. The relationship between the ethical principle of autonomy and the law of trespass to the person.			
2. The role of consent in healthcare.			
3. The elements of a valid consent.			
4. Decision-making capacity.			
5. The provisions for providing care and treatment to a person who lacks decision-making capacity.			

Where you are not confident in your knowledge of a topic, what will you do next?

Further reading

Department for Constitutional Affairs (2007) *Mental Capacity Act 2005 Code of Practice*. London: The Stationery Office.

Department of Health (2001) *Good Practice in Consent* (HSC 2001/023). London: The Stationery Office.

Ministry of Justice (2008) Deprivation of liberty: Code of Practice to supplement the main Mental Capacity Act 2005 Code of Practice. London: TSO.

Useful websites

www.dh.gov.uk Department of Health. Good range of information on consent including model consent forms.

www.justice.gov.uk Ministry of Justice. Detailed legal guidance on the Mental Capacity Act 2005.

www.nres.npsa.nhs.uk National Research Ethics provides up-to-date information concerning ethical research in healthcare.

Chapter 5

Mental health and the law

NMC Standards of Proficiency

This chapter will address the following NMC *Standards of Proficiency* and *Outcomes to be achieved for entry to the branch programme.*

Practise in accordance with an ethical and legal framework which ensures the primacy of patient and client interest and well-being and respects confidentiality.

Outcomes to be achieved for entry to the branch programme:
Demonstrate an awareness of legislation relevant to nursing practice:

- identify key issues in relevant legislation relating to mental health.

Chapter aims

By the end of this chapter you will be able to:

- state the principles of the Mental Health Act 1983;
- describe the requirements for compulsory admission;
- outline the key detention provisions of the Mental Health Act 1983;
- evaluate the safeguards designed to protect patients undergoing treatment for a mental disorder;
- discuss the arrangements for the rehabilitation and aftercare of patients detained for treatment.

Introduction

The position of the patient with mental health problems is now more legalised than ever before (Unsworth, 1987). In addition to the provisions of the Mental Health Act 1983, a strong body of case law has developed that deals with fundamental issues of liberty, autonomy and respect.

When caring for a person with mental health problems, it is essential that as a nurse you not only apply the requirements of the legislation accurately but that you do so ethically and with due regard for the patient's rights. To assist you the Mental Health Act 1983 is accompanied by a Code of Practice that offers guidance on the application of the law (DH, 1999a). The code, if followed, will allow you to show clearly that you have discharged your duties by applying the law in a transparent, ethical and respectful way.

The Mental Health Act 1983

In England and Wales, mental healthcare is regulated through the provisions of the Mental Health Act 1983 as amended by the Mental Health Act 2007.

Despite a long-standing policy of community-focused service delivery and support, the legislation continues to centre on:

- entry into,
- care in, and
- discharge from institutions.

The fundamental aim of the 1983 Act is to strengthen the rights of patients made subject to its compulsory powers. This is achieved through five key principles that all have a liberal thrust:

- Increased recourse to review of detention.
- Enhanced civil and social status.
- Ideology of terminology.
- Least restrictive alternative.
- Multidisciplinary review of medical conditions.

Increased recourse to review of detention

Detention in hospital has been limited by time since the Lunacy Act 1890. Detained patients have a right to appeal against detention through the Mental Health Review Tribunal (MHRT), which considers whether the criteria for detention continue to be met.

A right of appeal for those detained for assessment was introduced for the first time by the Mental Health Act 1983.

Scenario 5.1

Discharge by a Mental Health Review Tribunal

In *R (on the application of C) v Secretary of State for the Home Department* [2002], the Court of Appeal dismissed an application by the Home Secretary calling for a decision to discharge a patient by the MHRT to be quashed.

The Court of Appeal held that the MHRT had heard evidence that the patient no longer met the detention conditions of the Mental Health Act 1983 and would therefore be discharged.

To ensure that all detained patients have their case independently reviewed, hospital managers now have a duty to refer a case to the MHRT where the patient has not appealed and remains detained in hospital for six months following their admission (Mental Health Act 1983, section 68).

Hospital managers are also empowered to conduct their own reviews of detention and order discharge where three or more agree that the detention conditions are not met (Mental Health Act 1983, section 23).

Scenario 5.2

Discharge can only be ordered where three or more managers agree

In *R (Tagoe-Thompson) v Central and North West London Mental Health NHS Trust*
[2002], a man suffering from paranoid schizophrenia appealed to the hospital
managers against his detention for treatment under section 3 of the Mental Health
Act 1983.

Three managers met to review the detention and two agreed that the patient
should be discharged. However, as one of the panel objected, the court agreed that
the patient could not be discharged as the requirement of section 23 of the Mental
Health Act 1983, giving the power of discharge to the hospital managers, required
it to be exercised by three or more people.

Enhanced civil and social status

This principle was advocated mainly on therapeutic rather than legal grounds. One way
the law was able to implement this principle was through the right to vote. Informal in-
patients were given the right to vote by allowing them to register their entitlement using
a previous address (Representation of the People Act 1983).

Detained patients did not gain the right to vote until an amendment to the House of
Lords Reform Act 2001 granted it subject to the patient's capacity to decide.

Ideology of entitlement

This principle promoted the concept of access to services as a legal right. Patients who
have been detained for treatment are entitled to aftercare services as a right.

There is a duty on the health and social services to continue to provide aftercare
until it appears to them that the patient is no longer in need of that service (Mental
Health Act 1983, section 117). The duty is owed to individual patients who cannot be
charged for the aftercare services.

Scenario 5.3

Aftercare is a duty owed to individual patients

In *R (on the application of Stennett) v Manchester City Council* [2002], patients who
had been discharged from hospital after detention for treatment for a mental
disorder complained to the court that they were required to pay for their stay in a
care home. The House of Lords held that the provision of aftercare was a right owed
to patients detained for treatment under the Mental Health Act 1983, section 117.
The local authority and the health service were not entitled to ask patients to pay
for that aftercare and so their care home fees would have to be reimbursed.

Least restrictive alternative

Any use of formal powers under the 1983 Act must be the least restrictive means of
meeting the needs of the patient. The Approved Mental Health Professional (AMHP; see
page 98) has a duty to ensure that the person is actively resisting admission to hospital
and that compulsory admission is the most appropriate method of dealing with the case.

The AMHP must also certify that the detention order used is the least restrictive
method of meeting the needs of the patient.

Multidisciplinary review of medical decisions

When formal admission under the Mental Health Act 1983 is considered, this falls to the AMHP whose role is to ensure that the person appears to be suffering from a mental disorder that warrants compulsory confinement. This initial safeguard ensures that people who do not have a mental disorder or those who do not actively resist admission are not improperly detained.

Further multidisciplinary reviews of medical decisions occur under part 4 of the 1983 Act, which provides safeguards concerning consent to treatment in certain cases. For example, patients who are subject to the consent to treatment provisions have a legal right to be supported through the treatment process by an Independent Mental Capacity Advocate (Mental Health Act 1983, section 130A).

The Mental Health Act Commission is an independent watchdog that oversees the implementation of the 1983 Act, and safeguards and promotes the rights of patients subject to the Act's compulsory powers. They make both announced visits and unannounced inspections of every mental health facility in order to:

- keep under review the operation of the Mental Health Act 1983 in respect of patients detained or liable to be detained under that Act;
- visit and interview, in private, patients detained under the Mental Health Act in hospitals and mental nursing homes;
- consider the investigation of complaints where these fall within the Commission's remit;
- appoint registered medical practitioners and others to give second opinions in cases where this is required by the Mental Health Act;
- publish and lay before Parliament a report every two years;
- monitor the implementation of the Code of Practice and propose amendments to Ministers.

Scope of the Mental Health Act 1983

Part 1, section 1 of the Mental Health Act 1983 makes it clear that the Act shall have effect with respect to *the reception, care and treatment of mentally disordered patients, the management of their property and other related matters*. From the outset it is clear that the 1983 Act only applies to people who suffer from a mental disorder.

Definition of mental disorder

Mental disorder is the legal term used by the 1983 Act to establish who can be made subject to its provisions. It is defined as:

> *Any disorder or disability of the mind.*
>
> (Mental Health Act 1983, section 1(2))

As the definition is very broad, two safeguards are included to narrow the scope of the 1983 Act. A person with a learning disability cannot be compulsorily admitted for treatment or guardianship unless their disability is associated with abnormally aggressive or seriously irresponsible conduct (Mental Health Act 1983, section 1(2A)). Furthermore, dependence alone on alcohol or drugs cannot be considered a mental disorder for the purpose of the Act (Mental Health Act 1983, section 1(3)).

Scenario 5.4

The Mental Health Act 1983 only applies to the care and treatment of a person's mental disorder

In *St George's Healthcare NHS Trust v S* [1998], a pregnant woman with pre-eclampsia was detained under section 2 of the Mental Health Act 1983 when she refused hospital treatment for this life-threatening physical condition. The court held that her detention was unlawful because she did not have a mental disorder and the 1983 Act cannot be used to detain someone just because their thinking seemed unusual, irrational or contrary to public opinion. The Mental Health Act 1983 can only be used to justify detention for mental disorder.

Principles of compulsory detention

The process of detention aims to ensure that the only people made subject to the compulsory provisions of the 1983 Act are those who:

- are or appear to be suffering from a mental disorder; and
- are actively resisting admission to hospital.

In all other cases, informal admission under the provisions of section 131 of the Mental Health Act 1983 is more appropriate.

Deprivation of liberty

Compulsory detention means that a person is deprived of their liberty. Detention on the grounds that a person is suffering from a mental health problem is not in itself unlawful. As long as it is in accordance with the law, it will comply with the European Convention on Human Rights (Council of Europe, 1950). As specified in *Winterwerp v The Netherlands* (1979), the law must show that:

- unless it is an emergency,
- the person is reliably shown by objective medical evidence to be suffering from a mental disorder, and
- the disorder is of a nature or degree that warrants continued compulsory confinement.

Activity 5.1

Detention conditions

Look at the requirements for detention for each of the powers detailed in Appendix 5.1 (see pages 108–9). Do these requirements meet the conditions specified by the European Court of Human Rights in *Winterwerp v The Netherlands* (1979)?

An outline answer is given at the end of the chapter.

Compulsory admission

The detention process is a division of responsibility between three key people:

- the Approved Mental Health Professional;
- a registered medical practitioner; and
- the patient's nearest relative.

Approved Mental Health Professionals

Approved Mental Health Professionals (AMHPs) include nurses and social workers who have been approved by the local authority as having appropriate competence in dealing with people who have mental disorder (Mental Health Act 1983, section 114).

The AMHP generally makes the application for detention once they are satisfied that the person is suffering from a mental disorder and is actively resisting admission to hospital and has a duty to conduct a suitable interview with the person before making the application. The AMHP provides a safeguard against the misuse of detention powers and cannot be directed by their local authority or employer to apply for a person's detention.

Registered medical practitioners

Reliable, objective medical evidence is a fundamental requirement of lawful detention and an application for detention must be founded upon two medical recommendations (one in an emergency). One doctor must also be an approved clinician recognised by the Primary Care Trust as being competent in the diagnosis of mental disorder. This requirement meets the need for objective medical evidence under human rights law (MHA 1983, section 12).

The medical recommendation must also indicate that the person is suffering from a mental disorder of a nature or degree that warrants continued compulsory confinement.

The degree of the disorder is its current severity. The nature of the disorder is its prognosis and the person's past history, including previous admissions and compliance with treatment. Only one of these criteria needs to be satisfied to meet the requirements for detention.

Scenario 5.5

Nature or degree of the disorder warrants compulsory confinement

In R v Mental Health Review Tribunal for South Thames Region Ex p. Smith [1998], a patient appealed against his detention when he was returned to hospital having been absent without leave for a year with no medical intervention. While the court agreed that the degree of his disorder did not warrant detention, the nature of his disorder, which had been shown to have deteriorated rapidly and because of which he became a danger to the public by making explosive devices, did warrant his continued confinement.

The nearest relative

The nearest relative is a statutory friend allocated to a detained patient. The person is drawn from a hierarchy of relatives set out under section 26 of the 1983 Act, with the person in the highest category becoming the nearest relative unless someone lower down the list:

- ordinarily resides with the patient; or
- cares for the patient.

Where there are two or more people in the same category, the older person will be the nearest relative.

Scenario 5.6

A person who ordinarily resides with or cares for the patient

In *Dewen v Barnet Healthcare Trust and Barnet London Borough Council* [2000], a man detained for treatment under the Mental Health Act 1983 argued that his son, not his daughter, should be his nearest relative as he was older than his sister. He also argued that his detention was unlawful as his son would have objected to his detention.

The court held that, although the son would normally be regarded as the nearest relative, being the older of two people in the same category, his sister took precedence as nearest relative because she provided care on a regular basis for her father. She had agreed to his detention for treatment of his paranoid schizophrenia and so the detention was lawful.

The hierarchy of nearest relative means:

- husband, wife or civil partner;
- son or daughter;
- mother or father;
- brother or sister;
- grandparent;
- grandchild;
- uncle or aunt;
- nephew or niece;
- a person who is not a relative, but with whom the patient has been living for not less that five years.

The purpose of the nearest relative is to provide a statutory friend for the detained patient, and that person has the power to:

- make applications to admit a person under compulsion; where the AMHPs make the application they have to take reasonable steps to inform the nearest relative about an application, and are required to have regard to any wishes expressed by the nearest relative;
- veto an application for treatment (section 3) and guardianship (section 7);
- be given information by the hospital managers about the patient's detention and discharge unless the patient objects;
- discharge their relative from detention by giving 72 hours notice to an authorised person at the hospital; the discharge can be barred by the responsible clinician and a further application cannot be made for six months; the nearest relative then has 28 days to make an application to a Mental Health Review Tribunal for discharge;
- apply to the Tribunal for discharge in respect of a patient detained by a criminal court under section 37 of the Act;
- have the right to be involved in any consideration as to the aftercare needs of a patient unless the patient objects;
- make a formal complaint to the hospital managers and the Mental Health Act Commission.

A nearest relative may be removed by the County Court if they act unreasonably or are otherwise unsuitable. The patient, another relative, a person living with the patient or an AMHP can apply to have a nearest relative removed and replaced by the court (Mental Health Act 1983, section 29(2)).

Detention

The properly completed Mental Health Act forms are sufficient authority to detain the patient and convey them to the named hospital. Once in hospital the managers have a duty, usually delegated to a registered nurse, to inform the patient of the conditions of detention and their right to appeal or complain (Mental Health Act 1983, section 132).

Under the civil detention provisions a person can be detained either for assessment or for treatment. Where a person is detained for treatment, appropriate medical treatment must be available. This is defined as medical treatment appropriate to the patient's case, taking into account the nature and degree of the mental disorder and other circumstances of his or her case.

Scenario 5.7

In *Reid v United Kingdom* (2003) a patient argued that he was unlawfully detained as he was not having medical treatment. The court held that treatment could include control and supervision to prevent harm to himself or others because of his abnormally aggressive behaviour.

Informal admission

A person can enter hospital for assessment and treatment of their mental disorder without the need to be detained. Since 1959, formal admission to hospital has been reserved for those who actively resist admission. Informal admission is used for those who consent, those who are incapable of deciding on admission and those who come into hospital informally rather than be detained (Mental Health Act 1983, section 131).

A 16- or 17-year-old child must consent themselves to admission on an informal basis. Where the child lacks the capacity to make the decision or refuses admission on an informal basis, the decision cannot be made by a person with parental responsibility.

Holding powers

Informal patients who wish to leave hospital against medical advice can be made subject to the holding powers under section 5 of the 1983 Act (see Appendix 5.1, pages 108–9: Civil Detention Powers under the Mental Health Act 1983). The approved clinician or their nominated deputy may hold a patient for up to 72 hours to allow for an assessment to be made with a view to their detention under section 2 or section 3. Where the immediate attendance of an approved clinician cannot be secured, a nurse of the prescribed class may hold the person for up to six hours or until the clinician arrives on the ward (see Appendix 5.1).

For the purposes of the power to detain a patient in hospital for a maximum of six hours under section 5(4) of the Mental Health Act 1983 a nurse of the prescribed class is a first or second level registered nurse whose registration includes an entry indicating that the nurse's field of practice is either mental health or learning disabilities nursing (Mental Health (Nurses) (England) Order 2008 (SI 2008/1207))

Mentally disordered people who commit offences

Where a person commits an offence when suffering from a mental disorder, the Crown Prosecution Service and police must wherever possible divert the person away from the criminal justice system and arrange for the person's care and treatment (Crown Prosecution Service, 2004).

Even where prosecution is in the public interest, because of the seriousness of the crime, the courts have a range of options under the Mental Health Act 1983 to enable the person to be assessed and to receive care and treatment. Similarly, prison inmates who are in need of care and treatment can be transferred to hospital. These provisions are summarised in Appendix 5.2: Detention provisions for people with mental disorders who commit offences (pages 110–11).

Consent to treatment

Compulsory admission and treatment under the Mental Health Act 1983 are dealt with separately. Detention under the Act does not necessarily mean compulsory treatment. Section 56 of the Act specifically excludes most of the emergency provisions and holding powers from the consent to treatment provisions, including patients detained by virtue of:

- an emergency application (section 4);
- holding powers under sections 5(2) or (4);
- remand to hospital for a report on their mental condition (section 35);
- a detention by the police (sections 135 or 136);
- a detention in a place of safety (sections 37(4) or 45A(5)).

They also do not apply to a patient who is:

- conditionally discharged and not recalled to hospital (sections 42, 73 or 74);
- a community patient and not recalled to hospital (section 17A); or
- subject to guardianship (section 7).

The approved clinician

The care of a detained mental health patient is supervised by an approved clinician who is called the patient's responsible clinician. This person is not necessarily a consultant psychiatrist. Amendments introduced by the Mental Health Act 2007 have extended the professionals who can be appointed as approved clinicians to include consultant clinical psychologists, consultant nurses and occupational therapists.

The approved clinician will supervise the patient's treatment, grant leave and, where necessary, renew a detention order or discharge the patient from hospital (Mental Health Act 1983, sections 20 and 145).

Even though the provisions of the Mental Health Act 1983 allow for compulsory treatment without consent, it is essential that care and treatment are given in a climate of consent with respect for the rights and dignity of the patient. The European Convention on Human Rights places a negative obligation – a duty not to breach a patient's human rights – on mental health nurses. Treatment for mental disorder can engage rights under article 3: the right to be free from torture, inhuman and degrading treatment, and article 8: the right to respect for private and family life, which includes respect for personal autonomy and dignity.

Scenario 5.8

Treatment that is medically necessary is not inhuman or degrading

In *Herczegfalvy v Austria* (1993), the European Court of Human Rights held that mental healthcare called for increased vigilance in complying with the Convention. Nevertheless, as a general rule, a measure that is a therapeutic necessity cannot be regarded as inhuman or degrading. That is, the treatment must be in accordance with a responsible body of professional opinion and be in the patient's best interests.

In *R (on the application of PS) v RMO (DR G) and SOAD (DR W)* [2003], the court held that it was not a breach of article 8 of the Convention to require a patient detained for treatment to take medication for his mental disorder as it could be justified as necessary for the patient's health and for the protection of others from harm.

Treatment under the provisions of the Mental Health Act 1983 is defined as *nursing, psychological intervention and specialist mental health habilitation, rehabilitation and care*, the purpose of which is to *alleviate or prevent a worsening of the disorder or its symptoms* (Mental Health Act 1983, sections 145(1) and (4)). This recognises a treatment as a whole approach to mental disorder and allows for the treatment of a wide range of symptoms, including the force feeding of a patient refusing to eat and the taking of blood samples to monitor therapeutic levels of medication.

Compulsory treatment for a patient's mental disorder is allowed where it is given by, or under the direction of, the approved clinician.

Scenario 5.9

Force-feeding as treatment for mental disorder

In *B v Croydon HA* [1995], B, who suffered from a psychopathic disorder, was compulsorily detained in hospital under section 3 of the 1983 Act. One of her symptoms was a compulsion to harm herself. She stopped eating, with the result that her weight fell to a dangerous level, and it was decided to feed her by nasogastric tube. B went to court arguing that the health authority should not tube-feed her without her consent.

The court found that the word 'treatment' in section 63 of the 1983 Act referred to actions calculated to alleviate or prevent a deterioration of the mental disorder from which the patient was suffering. This included acts that prevented the patient from harming herself and so tube-feeding constituted treatment and could be carried out lawfully without B's consent.

Safeguards

Some treatment under the 1983 Act may only be given where provisions safeguarding patients have been met. There are three categories of safeguard.

- Treatments that require consent and a second opinion, including psychosurgery: these require both the consent of the patient and an agreeable second opinion from a doctor appointed by the Mental Health Act Commission (Mental Health Act 1983, section 57).

- Treatments that require consent or a second opinion, including the giving of medication for mental disorder beyond three months from when it was first administered: these require either the consent of the patient or an agreeable second opinion from an appointed doctor (Mental Health Act 1983, section 58).

In the case of electroconvulsive therapy (ECT):

- treatment cannot be given without the consent of a capable patient;
- treatment cannot be given without agreement from an appointed doctor where the person is incapable.

The second opinion appointed doctor will not be entitled to authorise ECT for an incapable patient where:

- there is a valid and applicable advance decision refusing ECT;
- an attorney with authority under an LPA refuses consent;
- a deputy with authority refuses consent.

(Mental Health Act 1983, section 58A)

The nurse as consultee

When asked to sanction treatment for a patient, second opinion appointed doctors must consult with two people, one a nurse and one who cannot be a doctor or a nurse, about the patient's condition.

Activity 5.2

The nurse's role as consultee

Imagine that you are to act as consultee for a patient whose treatment is being considered by a second opinion appointed doctor. Note down the topics you are likely to discuss with the doctor before they decide on the suitability of treatment for the patient.

Now read below for further information.

The nurse will have had direct knowledge of the person's history and condition, and be in a position to comment on the issues affecting the patient including:

- the proposed treatment and the patient's ability to consent to it;
- other treatment options;
- the way in which the decision to treat was arrived at;
- the facts of the case, progress, etc.;
- the view of the patient's relatives on the proposed treatment;
- the implications of imposing treatment upon a non-consenting patient;
- the reasons for the patient's refusal of treatment;
- any other matter relating to the patient's care on which the consultee wishes to comment.

Patients who initially consent to treatment may withdraw that consent. Treatment would have to cease unless it could be justified as urgent as set out in section 62.

Independent Mental Health Advocacy Service

An Independent Mental Health Advocacy (IMHA) service was established under the 1983 Act by an amendment introduced by the Mental Health Act 2007.

There is a duty to instruct an IMHA where a patient is a qualifying patient. A patient is a qualifying patient if they are:

- detained unthder the Mental Health Act (other than sections 4, 5(2), 5(4), 135 or 136);
- subject to guardianship; or
- a community patient; or
- discussing with a registered medical practitioner or approved clinician the possibility of being given treatment under section 57; or
- under 18 and not detained and discussing with a doctor or approved clinician the possibility of being given ECT.

The role of the IMHA is to help obtain information about and improve the patient's understanding of:

- the provisions of this Act;
- any conditions or restrictions to which he or she is subject;
- what (if any) medical treatment is given, proposed or discussed;
- why it is given, proposed or discussed;
- the authority under which it is, or would be, given; and
- the requirements of this Act which apply to giving the treatment to him or her.

To fulfil their role the IMHA may:

- visit and interview the patient in private;
- visit and interview the person professionally concerned with his or her medical treatment;
- require the production of and inspect any records relating to his or her detention or treatment or aftercare service and records held by a local social services authority which relate to him or her.

Rehabilitation and aftercare

Leave of absence

Testing a patient's response to treatment by allowing controlled periods away from hospital is an important element of the rehabilitation process. An approved clinician may grant a detained patient a leave of absence from hospital. The leave may be subject to any conditions the approved clinician considers necessary (Mental Health Act 1983, section 17). The period of leave is at the responsible clinician's discretion and can range from hours to seven days, or longer if the use of a community treatment order is deemed unsuitable. A patient may be recalled to hospital if they do not fulfil the conditions set out when the leave was granted, without the need to undergo a new detention application.

Community treatment orders

Where long-term leave of over seven days is contemplated, the responsible clinician must first consider the use of a community treatment order. This order allows an approved clinician to test the rehabilitation of a patient detained for treatment by discharging the patient subject to their being recalled to hospital if they do not continue with treatment in the community.

A patient subject to a community treatment order is known and referred to in law as a *community patient*. A community patient cannot be made to take treatment by force in the community. Where compulsory treatment is deemed necessary, recall to hospital would be necessary.

The responsible clinician may make a community treatment order for a patient detained under the Mental Health Act 1983 for treatment under sections 3, 47 and 48 of the 1983 Act, if they are satisfied that the following criteria are met and an AMHP agrees that a community treatment order is appropriate for that patient.

- The patient must need medical treatment for their mental disorder for their own health or safety, or for the protection of others.
- It must be possible for the patient to receive the treatment they need without having to be in hospital.
- The patient may be recalled to hospital for treatment should this become necessary.
- Appropriate medical treatment for the patient must be available while living in the community.
- The responsible clinician must state the conditions of the order that have been agreed with the AMHP.
- Where the patient does not comply with the conditions, this can be taken into account when considering a recall to hospital.
- The responsible clinician may also recall a community patient to hospital if:
    o they require medical treatment in hospital for mental disorder; and
    o there would be a risk of harm to the health or safety of the patient or to other persons if they were not recalled to hospital for that purpose.

Aftercare

Patients detained for treatment under the Mental Health Act 1983 have a right to aftercare under section 117 of the Act. It is the duty of the health and social services to provide any aftercare services they consider necessary for the patient. As aftercare is a right, the services provided cannot be charged for. The provision of aftercare must continue as long as the health and social services consider the patient requires it. The decision to end aftercare services must be a joint one.

Scenario 5.10

Aftercare is an individual right owed to a patient discharged after a period of detention for treatment

In *R v Ealing District HA Ex p. Fox* [1993], a man successfully argued that his health authority had breached its duty to provide aftercare when it accepted that its doctors did not wish to care for the patient.

The court held that the health authority had not discharged its statutory obligations by merely accepting its own doctors' opinions. It had a duty to make arrangements itself with other health authorities or the private sector; if it failed, it should have referred the matter back to the Secretary of State for Health.

Guardianship

Under the Mental Health Act 1983, section 7, guardianship provides an alternative to detention for compulsory treatment by requiring a person with a mental disorder to:

- live at an address specified by the Guardian;
- provide access to people named by the Guardian, such as a doctor, nurse or social worker;
- attend any place the Guardian may specify for medical treatment, occupation, education or training.

No treatment may be given to the patient without consent. Guardianship is administered by the local social services authority. They will name a social worker as Guardian or accept a person known to the patient, such as a relative who is suitable and willing to act in the role.

The use of guardianship has been declining, despite the Mental Health Act Commission's attempt to encourage its use.

C H A P T E R   S U M M A R Y

- Mental healthcare is regulated through the provisions of the Mental Health Act 1983 as amended by the Mental Health Act 2007.
- The fundamental aim of the 1983 Act is to strengthen the rights of patients made subject to its compulsory powers through five key principles that all have a liberal thrust.
- The provisions of the Mental Health Act 1983 only apply to people who suffer from a mental disorder.
- Mental disorder is defined as any disorder or disability of the mind.
- Only people who are, or appear to be, suffering from a mental disorder and who actively resist admission to hospital are considered to be subject to compulsory powers under the 1983 Act.
- Approved Mental Health Professionals (AMHPs) include nurses and social workers who have been approved by the local authority as having appropriate competence in dealing with people who have mental disorders.
- Detained patients must be informed of the conditions of detention and their right to appeal or complain once in hospital and the managers usually delegate this duty to a registered nurse.
- A person can enter hospital for assessment and treatment of their mental disorder as an informal admission, without the need to be detained.
- Admission and treatment under the Mental Health Act 1983 are dealt with separately.
- Some treatment under the 1983 Act may only be given where provisions safeguarding patients have been met.
- An approved clinician may grant a detained patient a leave of absence from hospital.
- Where long-term leave, over seven days, is contemplated, the responsible clinician must first consider the use of a community treatment order.
- Guardianship provides an alternative to detention for treatment.
- The Code of Practice to the Mental Health Act 1983 provides clear guidance about your role and duties under the Act.
- The requirements of the Act and its Code of Practice must be followed to ensure that patients are cared for with respect and with due regard for their fundamental rights and freedoms.

Activities: brief outline answer

5.1 Detention conditions (page 97)

You will see that the detention conditions for compulsory admission do reflect the requirements of *Winterwerp v The Netherlands* (1979). For example, section 2 of the Mental Health Act 1983, Ordinary Admission for Assessment, requires that:

- the person is suffering from a mental disorder;
- of a nature or degree that warrants detention in hospital for assessment;
- in the interests of his own health or safety or protection of others;
- the application must be founded upon the recommendation of two doctors, one of whom must be recognised as having experience in the diagnosis and treatment of mental disorder under section 12 of the Mental Health Act 1983.

Knowledge review

Now that you've worked through the chapter, how would you rate your knowledge of the following topics?

	Good	Adequate	Poor
1. The principles of the Mental Health Act 1983.			
2. The requirements for compulsory admission.			
3. The key detention provisions of the Mental Health Act 1983.			
4. The safeguards designed to protect patients undergoing treatment for a mental disorder.			
5. The arrangements for the rehabilitation and aftercare of patients detained for treatment.			

Where you are not confident in your knowledge of a topic, what will you do next?

Further reading

Bartlett, P (2005) *Blackstone's Guide to The Mental Capacity Act 2005*. London: Oxford University Press.

Jones, R (2007) *Mental Health Act Manual*. London: Sweet and Maxwell.

Useful websites

www.dh.gov.uk/en/Policyandguidance/Healthandsocialcaretopics/Mentalhealth/index.htm Department of Health Mental Health Law page.

Appendix 5.1: Civil detention provisions under Mental Health Act 1983, part 2, as amended

Section no. and purpose	Method	Conditions for detention	Duration	Can the patient apply to MHRT?	Can nearest relative apply to MHRT?	Automatic MHRT referral?	Do consent to treatment rules apply?
Section 4: Emergency admission for assessment	Application by AMHP or nearest relative founded on one medical recommendation	As for section 2, but AMHP or nearest relative must certify that it is of urgent necessity for the patient to be admitted and complying with section 2 would involve undesirable delay	72 hours; can be converted to ordinary admission for assessment if a second medical recommendation is received during this time	No, but an appeal under section 2 can begin	No	No	No
Section 2: Ordinary admission for assessment	Application by AMHP founded on two medical recommendations, one of which is from an approved clinician	Person is suffering from mental disorder of a nature or degree that warrants the detention of the patient in a hospital for assessment (or for assessment followed by medical treatment) for at least a limited period; and person ought to be so detained in the interests of his or her own health or safety or with a view to the protection of other persons	28 days, not renewable; will be extended to the date of the hearing where a nearest relative is being displaced by the county court	Yes, within first 14 days	Yes	No	Yes
Section 3: Admission for treatment	Application by AMHP founded on two medical	Person is suffering from mental disorder of a nature or degree that makes it appropriate for them to	6 months; can be renewed under section 20 for a	Yes, within first 6 months,	Yes	Yes, if a completed	Yes

			further 6 months, then yearly	then once in each period of detention	appeal has not occurred in first 6 months
	recommendations, one of which is from an approved clinician	receive medical treatment in a hospital; and it is necessary for the health or safety of the patient or for the protection of other persons that they should receive such treatment; and it cannot be provided unless they are detained under this section; and appropriate medical treatment is available			
Section 5(2)	Report from a doctor or approved clinician in charge of the patient's treatment	In-patient in a hospital who appears to a registered medical practitioner or approved clinician in charge of their treatment to need detention under this part of this Act	72 hours, not renewable	No	No
Section 5(4)	Report from a nurse of the prescribed class	Appears to a nurse of the prescribed class that (a) a patient who is receiving treatment for mental disorder as an in-patient in a hospital is suffering from mental disorder to such a degree that it is necessary for his or her health or safety or for the protection of others for him or her to be immediately restrained from leaving the hospital; and (b) it is not practicable to secure the immediate attendance of a practitioner or clinician to furnish a report under section 5(2)	6 hours, not renewable	No	No

Appendix 5.2: Detention provisions for people with mental disorder who commit offences

Section no. and purpose	Duration	Application to MHRT?	Nearest relative application to MHRT?	Automatic referral to MHRT?	Do consent to treatment provisions apply?
Section 35: Remand to hospital for psychiatric report	28 days; may be renewed by the court for further periods of 28 days to a maximum of 12 weeks	No	No	No	No
Section 36: Remand to hospital for treatment	28 days; may be renewed by the court for further periods of 28 days to a maximum of 12 weeks	No	No	No	Yes
Section 37: Hospital order by the court	6 months, renewable for further 6 months, then yearly	In second 6 months, then in each period of detention	In second 6 months and then each period of detention	After 3 years if the patient remains in hospital and has not made an appeal of their own	Yes
Section 37: Guardianship order by the court	6 months, renewable for further 6 months then yearly	Within first 6 months, then in each period of detention	Within first year then yearly	No	No
Sections 37/41: Hospital order with restriction	Without limit of time; discharge and leave of absence restricted by the Home Office	In second 6 months, then in each period of detention	No nearest relative	If one has not been held, Home Secretary will refer the case to the MHRT every 3 years	Yes
Section 38: Interim hospital order	12 weeks; may be renewed in 28-day periods to a maximum of 1 year	No	No	No	Yes
Section 45A:	Without limit of time	In first 6 months,	No	Home secretary	Yes

Hospital and limitation direction		second 6 months, then yearly		will refer case every 3 years if one has not been held	
Section 46: Transfer to hospital of patient in custody during Her Majesty's pleasure	Without limit of time	Within first 6 months, then once in each period of detention	No	Home Secretary will refer case every 3 years if one has not been held	Yes
Section 47: Transfer to hospital of a person serving a prison sentence	6 months, a further 6 months, then a year at a time	Within first 6 months, then once in each period of detention	No	Hospital managers will refer case every 3 years if one has not been held	Yes
Sections 48/49: Transfer with restrictions	Restriction lapses on earliest release date from prison	In second 6 months after transfer, then yearly	No nearest relative	Home secretary will refer case every 3 years if one has not been held	Yes
Section 48: Transfer of other prisoners for urgent treatment	According to treatment needs of the patient	Within first 6 months, then once in each period of detention	No	Home Secretary will refer case every 3 years if one has not been held	Yes
Sections 48/49 Transfer with restriction	Restriction will lapse on earliest release date	In second 6 months, then each period of detention	No nearest relative	Home secretary will refer case every 3 years if one has not been held	Yes
Section 136: Police power in places to which the public have access	72 hours, not renewable	No	No	No	No
Section 135: Warrant to enter and search for a person with mental disorder	72 hours, not renewable	No	No	No	No

Chapter 6

Consent and children

Chapter aims

By the end of this chapter you will be able to:

* state the three developmental stages a child passes through to become an autonomous adult;
* outline how the law bestows parental responsibility for a child;
* describe the extent of a person with parental responsibility's right to consent to treatment for a child;
* analyse the test for Gillick competence;
* examine the requirements for a valid consent from a child who is 16 or 17 years old;
* judge when it is lawful to restrict a child's liberty in order to provide care and treatment.

Introduction

Nurses have patients of all ages and it is essential that any care or treatment delivered to them is done within the law. Consent is an essential element of the lawfulness of treatment. It provides a defence to criminal assault and the tort or civil wrong of trespass to the person (*F v West Berkshire HA* [1990]). Consent in a health context also has a more fundamental objective. Lord Mustill, in *Airedale NHS Trust v Bland* [1993], wondered why it was that doctors and nurses can with impunity perform acts on people that would be crimes if done by ordinary citizens. He held that:

> *The reason why the consent of the patient is so important is not that it furnishes a defence in itself, but because it is usually essential to the propriety of medical treatment.*
>
> (*Airedale NHS Trust v Bland* [1993], Lord Mustill at 889)

Unless a valid consent is present or consent is dispensed with by operation of law, such as in an emergency, the acts of nurses would lose their immunity.

The nature of consent

Consent is a state of mind in which a person agrees to the touching of their body as part of an examination or treatment (*Sidaway v Bethlem Royal Hospital* [1985]). It has a clinical and legal purpose. The clinical purpose recognises that the success of treatment depends very often on the cooperation of the patient. The legal purpose is to underpin the propriety of the treatment and furnish a defence to the crime and tort of trespass. For capable adults, the law recognises the right to self-determination, which includes the right to consent to or refuse medical treatment even if this would lead to their death.

Children reach the age of majority or adulthood at 18. However, while the courts acknowledge that no minor or child under 18 is a wholly autonomous being, they do recognise the right of the minor to consent to medical treatment as they develop and mature with age.

Consent and children

Kennedy and Grubb (1998) argue that children pass through three developmental stages on the journey to becoming fully autonomous adults:

- the child of tender years;
- the Gillick competent child;
- children 16 and 17 years old.

The child of tender years

Early Roman law allowed a father to literally have the power of life or death over his child. The overwhelming power a father had was gradually removed during the nineteenth century by Talfourd's Act, the Custody of Infants Act 1839 and the Matrimonial Causes Act 1857. Yet children were still seen to be in the custody of their parents, who retained considerable power over them. For example, parents could demand that a child in care be handed back when they were old enough to earn a wage (*Barnado v McHugh* [1891]).

The relationship between a child and a parent was formalised in the Children Act 1989. This Act allows parents to have parental responsibility for their children, which includes a right to consent to treatment.

Parental responsibility

The concept of parental responsibility replaced the notion of parental rights.

Parental responsibility is defined as all the rights, duties, powers, responsibility and authority that, by law, a parent of a child has in relation to the child and its property (Children Act 1989, section 2). These are not defined or specified in the Act. In essence, the Act empowers a person to make most decisions in a child's life, including consenting to medical treatment on the child's behalf.

Parental responsibility may be shared and generally decisions about a child can be made independently. In most cases, only the consent of one person with parental responsibility is needed to proceed with treatment.

Activity 6.1

Parental responsibility

- List all the people you think might have parental responsibility for a child.
- From that list select the person who you think would have automatic parental responsibility by law.

An outline answer is given at the end of the chapter.

Automatic parental responsibility

Parental responsibility is conferred automatically on the mother of the child and the father if he was married to the mother at the time of the birth (Children Act 1989, section 2). If unmarried parents subsequently marry, the child's father gains parental responsibility for his children (Family Law Reform Act 1987, section 1).

In recognition of the changing demographic of the family and to encourage both parents to play a full part in the upbringing of their child, the Children Act 1989 was amended in December 2003 to allow unmarried natural fathers to have automatic parental responsibility if they become registered as the child's father under any of the birth registration statutes from that date.

Acquired parental responsibility

If a father is not married to his child's mother and was not registered as the child's father from December 2003, he may still acquire parental responsibility under an agreement with the mother or by order of the court (Children Act 1989, section 3). Parental responsibility may also be acquired by others, such as those in possession of an emergency protection order or a care order, but only for the duration of the order.

Step-parents

Since December 2005, a step-parent who is married to a child's natural parent can acquire parental responsibility either by agreement with the natural parents or by order of the court (Children Act 1989, section 4A).

Delegation of parental responsibility

The Children Act 1989, section 2(9), allows a person with parental responsibility to arrange for someone else to exercise it on their behalf. This delegation need not be in writing and allows carers such as schools, nannies and childminders to make delegated decisions on behalf of a person with parental responsibility for the child. For example, a nurse may visit a young child to find him or her in the care of a grandmother. As long as the nurse is satisfied that the grandmother is acting with the authority of a person with parental responsibility, such as the child's mother, she may accept the grandmother's consent as permission to treat the child.

Carers

The Children Act 1989 allows those who have care for a child, but not parental responsibility, to do what is reasonable in all the circumstances to promote or safeguard the child's welfare (Children Act 1989, section 3(5)). In terms of medical treatment, what is reasonable would generally require the consent of a person with parental responsibility unless it was an emergency or the treatment was trivial.

The extent of parental responsibility

Although a person with parental responsibility can generally make decisions independently, the freedom of each to act alone is not unfettered.

The Court held in *Re J* [2000] that there is a small group of important decisions made on behalf of a child that should not be carried out or arranged by one parent alone, even though they have parental responsibility under the Children Act 1989.

Activity 6.2

Limits to parental responsibility

In relation to a child, what kind of decisions do you think should not be made by one parent alone? Please do not read the next part unless you want to know the answer.

Now read below for further information.

Where the agreement of each person with parental responsibility is not forthcoming, the decision must not be made without the specific approval of the court. As held in *Re B (A Child)* [2003], the important decisions include:

- sterilisation of a child;
- changing a child's surname;
- circumcision of a child;
- a hotly disputed immunisation.

Authority to intervene

In *KD (A Minor) (Ward: Termination of Access)* [1988], the House of Lords held that the best persons to bring up a child are the natural parents. Their view is that public authorities cannot improve on nature and parents are given the exclusive privilege of bringing up a child with the decisions of devoted and responsible parents being treated with respect.

However, a parent's right to consent is not absolute. Parents' rights exist only for the benefit of the child and must be exercised in the child's best interests. The courts, through their inherent jurisdiction, exercise a supervisory role over parental decision making and can overrule a parental decision that is not in the best interests of the welfare of the child.

Under the private law provisions of the Children Act 1989, section 8, the court also has the power to settle a dispute between two or more people with parental responsibility.

Private law is not a question of child protection and so the threshold criterion of significant harm does not have to be engaged for the court to have jurisdiction.

As long as there is a dispute between people regarding an issue of parental responsibility for a child, the court can intervene to settle the issue.

Private law orders

The Children Act 1989, section 8, gives the court powers to resolve disputes regarding an issue of parental responsibility for a child. The orders available are:

- **residence order**, which settles with whom a child should live and bestows parental responsibility on that person where necessary;
- **contact order**, which settles contact arrangements with a child; contact can be as widely interpreted as the court sees fit and ranges from telephone and email contact to visits and holidays;
- **prohibited steps order**, which prohibits an action without the permission of the court;
- **specific issues order**, which allows the court to settle a specific issue in relation to the parental responsibility of a child.

Where the health and welfare of a child are at issue, the courts have been prepared to use these orders in a creative way.

Scenario 6.1

Using a residence order to bestow parental responsibility

In *B v B (A Minor) (Residence Order)* [1992], a child lived with her grandmother at the request of her mother but found that the child's school and GP would not accept the grandmother's consent for such things as school outings and routine treatments such as immunisations. The court granted the grandmother a residence order, because the welfare of the child required her to have parental responsibility, even though where the child lived was not an issue.

Prohibited steps and specific issues orders are also used by the courts to settle issues concerning a child's healthcare. In *J (A Minor) (Prohibited Steps Order: Circumcision)* [2000], the English mother of J, aged five, was granted a prohibited steps order preventing his Muslim father from making arrangements to have him circumcised without a court order, because ritual circumcision was an irreversible operation that was not medically necessary and had physical and psychological risks, and in such cases the consent of both parents was essential.

Scenario 6.2

Authorising medical treatment through a specific issues order

In *Camden LBC v R (A Minor) (Blood Transfusion)* [1993], a child's parents refused to allow him to have a blood transfusion for the treatment of B-cell lymphoblastic leukaemia because of their religious beliefs. The court found that, where the life of a child was at risk, it was essential to act urgently. The private law requirements of the Children Act 1989, section 8, could be used to seek a specific issues order. This procedure allows the matter to be brought before a High Court judge, who could order the treatment without delay and without transferring parental responsibility.

Authorising treatment against the wishes of a child's parents is reserved for the most serious cases. In *A&D v B&E* [2003], the High Court accepted that, in general, there is wide scope for parental objection to medical intervention. The Court considers medical interventions as existing on a scale. At one end are obvious cases where parental objection would have no value in child welfare terms, for example urgent life-saving treatment such as a blood transfusion.

At the other end are cases where there is genuine scope for debate and the views of the parents are important. These would not raise questions of neglect or abuse that would trigger child protection proceedings. Although an NHS Trust can obtain leave to apply for a specific issues order (Children Act 1989, section 8) it is unlikely that leave would be granted in the face of unified parental opposition to this type of treatment.

Scenario 6.3

Urgent and non-urgent treatment

In *Re P (A Minor)* (1981), the court directed that a termination could proceed on a 15-year-old child despite the genuinely held objections of her parents on religious and other grounds.

In *Re B (A Child)* [2003], the Court of Appeal held that, while it was prepared to settle a dispute between two parents on the issue of childhood immunisations, it would not do so where the dispute was between a parent and the health authorities.

The best interests test

The right of a parent to exercise their right to consent to treatment for a child is subject to them acting in the child's best interests. The court is also required to act in the best interests of the welfare of a child whenever a case is brought before them. The test for determining the best interests of a child has developed as new cases have been brought to court for judgment.

In one of the earliest cases, the court limited its consideration of a best interest to the life expectancy of the child. In *Re B (A Minor) (Wardship: Medical Treatment)* [1981], a child born with Down's syndrome needed urgent surgery for an intestinal blockage. The parents took the view that it would be kinder to let the child die than to allow her to grow up as a physically and mentally handicapped person. The judge held that the surgery was straightforward and that, as the child was expected to live for 20 to 30 years, surgery was in her best interests.

Some ten years later the court refined the determination of a best interest to include pain and suffering. In *J (A Minor) (Child in Care: Medical Treatment)* [1993], a profoundly brain-damaged child with a very short life expectancy was not thought to be benefiting from treatment, and both the parents and medical team sought an order allowing them to curtail treatment.

In the child's interest the Official Solicitor argued that an absolutist test applied, that in the case of a child everything should be done to preserve the child's life right to the bitter end and a court was never justified in denying consent to treatment to save life.

The court held that the absolutist test never applied. The denial of treatment to prolong life could only be sanctioned where it was in the best interests of the patient, and the test applicable was that of the child's best interests in those circumstances, and that was based on an assessment of the child's quality of life, and their future pain and suffering in relation to the life-saving treatment.

The need to go to court

Where those with parental responsibility strongly oppose the giving or withholding of treatment by a health professional to a child, the matter will need to be referred to the court for a decision. Failing to seek the court's approval for a plan of care in these circumstances would be a breach of the child's right to respect for a private and family life under article 8 of the European Convention on Human Rights.

Scenario 6.4

The need to go to court

In *Glass v United Kingdom* [2004], a severely physically and mentally disabled child complained that the UK had violated his right to physical integrity under the European Convention on Human Rights 1950 (article 8).

On his readmission with respiratory failure, the hospital insisted that he was dying and that diamorphine should be given to relieve his obvious distress. His mother disagreed and objected to the proposed treatment in the belief that it would harm his chances of recovery. Despite her objection, diamorphine was administered, but his condition improved and he returned home.

The European Court of Human Rights upheld the complaint, as treatment contrary to his mother's wishes breached his right to physical integrity under article 8, and the hospital had failed to seek the High Court's approval for the proposed treatment.

Permissive declarations

When the court's approval for a plan of care is sought, the method used to authorise treatment is by way of a declaration. Here the court declares that the proposed treatment is lawful. A declaration is binding on the parties before the court and the health professionals are bound by its terms.

The courts are aware that the terms of a declaration may restrict a health professional's ability to exercise their clinical judgement when caring for a child. If a court declares that a child should have no antibiotic therapy, for example, it would be unlawful for the doctor or nurse to give antibiotics even if it would relieve the suffering of a child.

To avoid such situations the courts resort to the use of permissive declarations. In a permissive declaration the court authorises the withholding of certain treatment at the discretion of the team caring for the child. It allows treatment to be given where this is in the best interests of the child and also allows treatment, even life-sustaining treatment, to be withheld where it is not considered in the child's best interests.

Scenario 6.5

The permissive declaration

In *Re Wyatt (A Child) (Medical Treatment: Continuation of Order)* [2005], the intervention of the court was sought in respect of the medical treatment of a child whose condition had significantly deteriorated, in that she had developed an intermittent rasping cough and it was likely that she was suffering from a viral infection. Medical experts were of the opinion that the only intervention for her, if she continued to deteriorate, would be intubation and ventilation, but that it would

Scenario 6.5 continued

not be in her best interests as essentially it would be futile. The view of the parents was that, if she were ventilated, she would recover.

The court made it clear that, in the best interests of the child, the care team should be able to refrain from having to intervene by way of intubation and ventilation. The authority was granted by way of a permissive non-mandatory declaration so that, at the moment the decision arose, the medical authorities were required to use their best judgement in the child's best interests as to whether to withhold the treatment or not. Accordingly, a decision to desist would be lawful.

Consent to treatment for a child of tender years is provided by a person with parental responsibility for the child, usually a parent. However, the decision of the parent must be in the best interests of the welfare of the child and can be overridden by a court exercising its inherent jurisdiction to act in the child's best interests.

The Gillick competent child

The matter of whether a child under 16 has the necessary capacity to consent to medical examination and treatment was decided by the House of Lords in *Gillick v West Norfolk and Wisbech AHA* [1986]. In this case, a mother objected to Department of Health advice that doctors could give contraceptive advice and treatment to children under 16 without parental consent. The court held that a child under 16 had the legal capacity to consent to medical examination and treatment, including contraceptive treatment, if they had sufficient maturity and intelligence to understand the nature and implications of that treatment.

The test for Gillick competence

Activity 6.3

Gillick competence

Before reading the next part make a list of the factors you think should be taken into account when deciding whether a child has sufficient maturity and intelligence to make a healthcare decision.

Now read below for further information.

In determining whether a child has sufficient maturity and intelligence to make a decision, nurses need to take account of the child, their chronological, emotional and mental age, and their intellectual development, as well as their ability to reach a decision. The aim of the Gillick principle is to reflect the transition of a child to adulthood. The legal capacity to make decisions is conditional on the child's gradually acquiring maturity and the ability to make decisions. The degree of maturity and capacity therefore depends on the gravity of the decision. A relatively young child would have sufficient maturity and intelligence to be capable of consenting to a plaster on a small cut. Equally, a child who had the capacity to consent to dental treatment or the repair of broken bones may lack capacity to consent to more serious treatment (*Re R (A Minor) (Wardship Consent to Treatment)* [1992]).

Scenario 6.6

Gillick competence for life-saving treatment

In *Re L (Medical Treatment: Gillick Competence)* [1998], a critically injured 14-year-old Jehovah's Witness had refused to consent to life-saving medical treatment because it would involve blood transfusions. The hospital authority wanted to carry out the treatment without her consent. The question for the court was whether L was competent to withhold consent within the rule in Gillick.

The court found that, despite her maturity, L was still a child and her beliefs had been developed through her sheltered upbringing within the Jehovah's Witness community. She knew she would die without treatment but had not been informed of the likely nature of her death. She was not Gillick competent and it was in her best interests for the treatment to be carried out.

With regard to contraceptive advice and treatment, there is much to be understood by the child if they are to have capacity to consent. The practitioner giving the advice or treatment would need to be satisfied that not only was the advice understood, but that the child had sufficient maturity to understand what was involved. This would include moral and family questions, such as the future relationship with parents, longer-term problems associated with the emotion of pregnancy or its termination, and the health risks associated with sexual intercourse at a young age.

Where the practitioner giving the advice or treatment is satisfied that the child is Gillick competent, the consent of the child is as effective as that of an adult. This consent cannot be overruled by a parent.

Fraser guidelines

Giving contraceptive advice and treatment to a child under 16 years of age gives rise to a concern that a practitioner may be accused of procuring sexual intercourse with a child under 16 years, which is a criminal offence (Sexual Offences Act 2003). To protect nurses from such accusations, Lord Fraser in *Gillick* issued guidance to ensure that contraceptive advice and treatment was only given on clinical grounds. There might be exceptional cases when, in the interests of the child's welfare, a nurse might give contraceptive advice and treatment without the permission or even knowledge of the parents. You must be satisfied:

- that the girl understood the advice;
- that you could not persuade her to tell or allow you to tell her parents;
- that she was likely to have sexual intercourse with or without contraceptive treatment;
- that, unless she received such advice or treatment, her physical or mental health was likely to suffer;
- her best interests required such advice or treatment without the knowledge or consent of her parents.

It is essential that this guidance is followed in practice to avoid any possibility of criminal conduct.

The defence offered by Lord Fraser's guidance has been extended by the Sexual Offences Act 2003, section 13. This provides a defence against aiding, abetting or counselling a sexual offence if the purpose is to:

- protect the child from sexually transmitted infection;
- protect the physical safety of the child;
- protect the child from becoming pregnant;
- promote the child's emotional well-being by the giving of advice, unless the purpose is to obtain sexual gratification or to cause or encourage the relevant sexual act.

Scenario 6.7

Giving sex and contraceptive advice without the knowledge of parents

In *R (Axon) v Secretary of State for Health* [2006], the court held that there was no reason why the rule in *Gillick* should not apply to other proposed treatment and advice.

The approach of a health professional to a young person seeking advice and treatment on sexual issues without notifying his or her parents should be in accordance with Lord Fraser's guidelines. There was no infringement of the rights of a young person's parents if a health professional was permitted to withhold information relating to the advice or treatment of the young person on sexual matters.

Children 16 and 17 years old

Children who have attained the age of 16 years have a right to consent to medical examination and treatment by statute. The Family Law Reform Act 1969, section 8, provides that:

- the consent of a minor who has attained the age of 16 years to any surgical, medical or dental treatment, which, in the absence of consent, would constitute a trespass to his person, shall be as effective as it would be if he were of full age; and where a minor has by virtue of this section given an effective consent to any treatment it shall not be necessary to obtain any consent for it from his parent or guardian;
- in this section 'surgical, medical or dental treatment' includes any procedure undertaken for the purposes of diagnosis, and this section applies to any procedure (including, in particular, the administration of an anaesthetic), which is ancillary to any treatment as it applies to that treatment.

The provisions allow a child of 16 or 17 years to give consent as if they were of full age, that is, an adult. Where such consent is given, it is as effective as that of an adult. It cannot be overruled by the child's parent or guardian.

The courts have adopted a very narrow construction of the provisions of section 8 of the 1969 Act. A child to whom the provisions apply can only consent to treatment or examinations that are therapeutic or diagnostic (*Re W (A Minor)(Medical Treatment Court's Jurisdiction)* [1992]). It does not allow consent for the donation of organs or blood. Even the giving of blood samples is excluded (separate provision is made for these under section 21(2) of the Family Law Reform Act 1969).

Contraceptive advice and treatment is considered a legitimate and beneficial treatment under section 5 of the National Health Service Act 1977 and section 41 of the National Health Service (Scotland) Act 1978. Children who have attained 16 years can consent to contraceptive advice and treatment, including termination of pregnancy.

The assessment of the capacity of a 16- or 17-year-old child to consent to treatment would be in accordance with the provisions of the Mental Capacity Act 2005 and its code of practice.

Activity 6.4

What happens if a child refuses consent to treatment?

You will have gathered so far that a competent child under 18 years can make treatment decisions and consent to treatment even though the person with parental responsibility objects. Imagine that the same competent child decides to refuse to consent to treatment. Discuss in a group the rights of the competent child to refuse treatment and what action can be taken when such a refusal happens. During the discussion, please make some notes of the issues raised.

An outline answer is given at the end of the chapter.

Parents and consent

Although both the courts and Parliament allow children to make treatment decisions for themselves as they mature, no minor, that is a child under 18 years, is a wholly autonomous being (Re M (A Child) (Refusal of Medical Treatment) [1999]). If a child under 18 refuses medical examination or treatment, the law does allow others to consent even if the child has capacity. Lord Donaldson summed up the position thus:

> I now prefer the analogy of the legal 'flak jacket' which protects you from claims by the litigious whether you acquire it from your patient, who may be a minor over the age of 16 or a 'Gillick competent' child under that age, or from another person having parental responsibilities which include a right to consent to treatment of the minor.
>
> Anyone who gives you a flak jacket (ie consent) may take it back, but then you only need one and so long as you continue to have one you have the legal right to proceed.
>
> (Re W (A minor)(Medical Treatment Court's Jurisdiction) [1992], Lord Donaldson MR at 641)

Where a child with capacity consents to medical examination or treatment, it cannot be overruled by a parent. However, where the same child refuses to consent, you may obtain it from another person with parental responsibility who has the right to consent to treatment on the child's behalf. (Note the exception to this rule under Mental Health Act 1983, section 131.)

Activity 6.5

Restricting a child's liberty

You may come across a situation where a competent child under 18 years refuses to remain in hospital. Discuss in a group what actions can be taken in such a situation. Make a note of the key points arising from your discussion.

Now read below for further information.

There may be occasions where a child refuses to remain in hospital for treatment. The Children Act 1989, section 25, allows the use of secure accommodation to restrict the liberty of a child.

Secure accommodation is not defined by the Children Act 1989. It depends on what use is made of the environment to restrict the liberty of a child, rather than having a pre-designated secure area. For example, locking the entrance to a ward, standing in a doorway or preventing a child leaving a room would be using accommodation in a secure way (*Re B (A Minor) (Treatment and Secure Accommodation)* [1997]).

The provisions of the Children Act 1989, section 25, apply to local authority homes, residential and nursing homes, and health and educational premises. The Act allows restriction without a court order for 72 hours in any 28-day period. A record must be kept of the nature and duration of the restriction. Where the period of restriction is going to be longer, a court order is required.

Conditions

Before restricting the liberty of a child you must be satisfied that he or she is 13 or older and has:

- a history of absconding and is likely to abscond from any other description of accommodation; and
- if they abscond they are likely to suffer significant harm; or
- if they are kept in any other description of accommodation they are likely to injure themselves or other persons.

Scenario 6.8

Restricting the liberty of a child

In *Re B (A Minor) (Treatment and Secure Accommodation)* [1997], a 17-year-old child suffered from a cocaine/crack addiction and was pregnant. Complications developed in the pregnancy that were potentially fatal to the patient and to the foetus.

However, B had a phobia about needles, doctors and any medical treatment, and wished to discharge herself from hospital. The hospital applied to the court for an order restricting her liberty by locking the door to the ward.

The court allowed the restriction of liberty and held that, while B had a right to refuse to give consent to medical treatment as she was over 16 years, that right could be overridden by the court or a person with parental responsibility for her. B's refusal carried little weight as it had been demonstrated that she could neither comprehend and retain information about her treatment, nor believe such information, and was unable to make a reasoned choice about her treatment.

The local authority and her mother having parental responsibility could take steps to protect her best interests, which could permit the use of reasonable force in order to administer the correct treatment.

The restriction of liberty was the essential factor in determining whether accommodation could be secure accommodation within the meaning of section 25 of the Children Act 1989, so that secure accommodation did not need to be previously designated but that each case would depend on its facts.

C H A P T E R   S U M M A R Y

- Consent is a state of mind in which a person agrees to the touching of their body as part of an examination or treatment.
- The courts acknowledge that no child under 18 is a wholly autonomous being.
- But the law recognises the right of a child to consent to medical treatment as they develop and mature with age.
- Children pass through three developmental stages to becoming a fully autonomous adult: the child of tender years, the Gillick competent child and the 16- and 17-year-old child.
- A person with parental responsibility is generally entitled to consent to treatment on behalf of a child.
- There is a small group of important decisions made on behalf of a child that should not be carried out or arranged by one parent alone.
- Parents' rights exist only for the benefit of the child and must be exercised in the child's best interests.
- Where those with parental responsibility strongly oppose the giving or withholding of treatment by a health professional to a child, the matter will need to be referred to the court for a decision.
- The court may use a permissive declaration to authorise the withholding of certain treatment at the discretion of the team caring for the child.
- A child under 16 has the legal capacity to consent to medical examination and treatment if they have sufficient maturity and intelligence to understand the nature and implications of that treatment.
- Children who have attained the age of 16 have a right to consent to medical examination and treatment under the Family Law Reform Act 1969, section 8.
- If a child under 18 refuses medical examination or treatment, the law does allow others to consent even if the child has capacity.
- Where a child with capacity consents to medical examination or treatment, it cannot be overruled by a parent.
- There may be occasions when a child refuses to remain in hospital for treatment and the Children Act 1989, section 25, can be used to restrict the liberty of a child.

Activities: brief outline answers

6.1 Parental responsibility (page 114)

Parental responsibility is defined as the rights duties, powers duties and responsibilities which by law a parent has in relation to a child (Children Act 1989, section 3):

- mother has automatic parental responsibility on the birth of the child (Children Act 1989, sections 2(1) and (2));
- father has parental responsibility if he was married to the child's mother at the time of the birth (Children Act 1989, section 2(1)); or
- if he subsequently married the mother of his child (Children Act 1989, section 2(3) & Family Law Reform Act 1987, section 1); or

- if he became registered as the father of the child after 30 December 2003 (Children Act 1989, section 4(1)(a)); or
- he and the child's mother make a parental responsibility agreement (Children Act 1989, section 4 (1)(b)).

That is made and recorded in the form prescribed by the Lord Chancellor;

or

- the Court on his application orders that he shall have parental responsibility (Children Act 1989, section 4(1)(c); or
- he obtains a residence order (Children Act 1989, section 12 read with section 4); or
- he is appointed as the child's guardian and the appointment takes effect (Children Act 1989, section 5).

Others who can acquire parental responsibility

- Step-parent if they are married to a parent with parental responsibility by agreement of the parents or order of the court.
- A person in possession of a residence order which could include the father of the child (Children Act 1989, section 12).
- A person appointed as the child's guardian once the appointment takes effect; this could include the father of the child (Children Act 1989, section 5).
- A person, other than a police officer, who is in possession of an emergency protection order (Children Act 1989 section 44(4)(c)).
- A person who has adopted a child (Adoption Act 1976, section 12 or Adoption & Children Act 2002, section 46).

A local authority may additionally acquire parental responsibility

- By obtaining a care order (Children Act 1989, section 31).
- By obtaining a freeing for adoption order (Adoption Act 1976, section 18) or a placement order (Adoption & Children Act 2002, section 21).

6.4 What happens if a child refuses consent to treatment? (page 122)

- No child under 18 years is wholly autonomous.
- If a child under 18 years refuses medical examination or treatment, the law does allow others to consent even if the child has capacity.
- Where a child with capacity consents to medical examination or treatment, it cannot be overruled by a parent.
- However, where the same child refuses to consent, you may obtain it from another person with parental responsibility who has the right to consent to treatment on the child's behalf.

Knowledge review

Now that you've worked through the chapter, how would you rate your knowledge of the following topics?

	Good	Adequate	Poor
1. The three developmental stages a child passes through to become an autonomous adult.			
2. How the law bestows parental responsibility for a child.			
3. The extent of a person with parental responsibility's right to consent to treatment for a child.			
4. The test for Gillick competence.			
5. The requirements for a valid consent from a child who is 16 or 17 years old.			
6. The requirements for the lawful restriction of a child's liberty in order to provide care and treatment.			

Where you are not confident in your knowledge of a topic, what will you do next?

Further reading

Griffith, R (2007) Changing families means changing parental responsibility. *BJM* 15(10): 654–5.

Griffith, R and Tengnah, C (2007) Protecting children: the role of the law 1. *BJCN* 12(3): 122.

Griffith, R and Tengnah, C (2007) Protecting children: the role of the law 2. *BJCN* 12(4): 175.

Useful websites

www.dh.gov.uk Department of Health.

www.opsi.gov.uk Children Act 1989.

www.unicef.org UN Convention on the rights of the child.

Chapter 7

Safeguarding children

NMC Standards of Proficiency

This chapter will address the following NMC *Standards of Proficiency* and *Outcomes to be achieved for entry to the branch programme.*

Practise in accordance with an ethical and legal framework which ensures the primacy of patient and client interest and well-being and respects confidentiality.

Outcomes to be achieved for entry to the branch programme:
Demonstrate an awareness of legislation relevant to nursing practice – identify key issues in relevant legislation relating to children.

Contribute to public protection by creating and maintaining a safe environment of care through the use of quality assurance and risk management strategies.

Outcomes to be achieved for entry to the branch programme:
Contribute to the identification of actual and potential risks to patients, clients and their carers, to oneself and to others:

• recognise and report situations that are potentially unsafe for patients and others.

Chapter aims

By the end of this chapter you will be able to:

• describe the five principles of the Children Act 1989;
• define significant harm;
• explain the role of the nurse in protecting children;
• describe the powers available to safeguard children from abuse.

Introduction

The United Nations Convention on the Rights of the Child (United Nations, 1989) requires the government to have regard to the full spectrum of human rights for all children and to consider children in legislative and policy decisions. The Convention defines a child as a person under the age of 18 years. In the UK the age of majority, at which a person reaches adulthood, was reduced from 21 to 18 years by the Family Law Reform Act 1969. People under 18 are often referred to in law as minors.

Article 19 of the United Nations Convention says that children have the right to be protected from abuse and the UK provides this protection through the Children Act 1989.

Nurses have a key role in the identification of children who may have been abused or who are at risk of abuse. They are also well placed to recognise when parents or other adults have problems that might affect their capacity to fulfil their roles with children safely.

Nurses must know when to refer a child for help as a 'child in need' (Children Act 1989, section 17) and how to act on concerns that a child is at risk of significant harm through abuse or neglect (Children Act 1989, section 31(10)).

Child abuse

Activity 7.1

The extent of child abuse

Before you continue to read the rest of this chapter, look at the annual summary of the most up-to-date child protection register statistics for England, Northern Ireland, Wales and Scotland (www.nspcc.org.uk). You do not need to read the whole document, just look at some of the key statistics to give you an idea of the extent of child abuse in the UK and the nature of the abuse.

Now read below for further information.

An estimated 300 million children worldwide are subjected to violence, exploitation and abuse. In Europe in 2003, the United Nations Children's Fund (2003) reported that two children die from abuse and neglect every week in Germany and the UK, and three a week in France. In the UK available figures show that there are 32,100 children on child protection registers as being at risk of abuse (Creighton, 2006).

A child protection register is a list of children who are at risk of abuse. The register acts as an alert that these children need special consideration.

Activity 7.2

Forms of abuse

Note down what you consider abuse to mean. Make a list of the types of activity with children that you would consider to be abusive.

Now read below for further information.

The following are the categories of abuse listed on the registers.

- **Neglect** – the persistent failure to meet a child's basic physical and/or psychological needs, which is likely to result in the serious impairment of the child's health or development.

Scenario 7.1

Neglect of a child

In *R v Banu* [1995], the parents of a child were jailed for three years after they admitted neglect as they had starved the child of adequate nourishment over a period of four months.

- **Physical abuse** – involves hitting, shaking, throwing, poisoning, burning, scalding, drowning, suffocating or causing other physical harm to a child.

Scenario 7.2

Physical abuse

In *R v Barraclough* [1992], a mother was sentenced to two years' detention for repeated attacks on her young child that resulted in a fractured skull.

- **Sexual abuse** – involves forcing or enticing a child or young person to take part in sexual activities. The activities may involve physical contact or non-contact activities such as those in Scenario 7.3.

Scenario 7.3

Sexual abuse

In *R v G* [1999], a brother received a jail sentence of seven years for the persistent sexual abuse of his sisters in the form of indecent assaults and rape.
    And in *R v B* [2001], a man was sentenced to nine months' imprisonment for taking indecent photographs of a child.

- **Emotional abuse** – persistent emotional ill treatment of a child such as to cause severe and persistent adverse effects on the child's emotional development.

Scenario 7.4

Emotional abuse

In *Re B (Children) (Emotional Welfare: Interim Care Order)* [2002], the Court of Appeal upheld an interim care order on two children on the grounds of emotional abuse when their father had made persistent threats to their lives during an acrimonious period of separation from their mother.

The category of concern is important as it requires nurses to identify evidence of a risk of significant harm before a child's name is placed on the register. In *R v Hampshire County Council* [1999], the Court of Appeal held that, before a child was placed on the child protection register there had to be evidence of significant harm, or a risk of such harm, in relation to the category of abuse under which the child was to be registered. For emotional abuse, nurses would have to be satisfied on the evidence before them that a child is at risk of suffering persistent or severe emotional ill-treatment or rejection. It is not enough to identify a stressful family situation – there must be evidence of a risk of significant harm to the child.

The Children Act 1989

The aim of the Children Act 1989 was to provide an effective legal framework for the safety and protection of children and it enshrines five main principles.

1. The welfare principle.
2. Keeping the family together.
3. The non-intervention principle.
4. Avoidance of delay.
5. Unified laws and procedures.

The welfare principle

The welfare principle states that, when a court determines any question with respect to the upbringing of a child or the child's property, the child's welfare shall be the court's paramount consideration (Children Act 1989, section 1).

Activity 7.3

Defining key terms

'Welfare' and 'paramount' are two terms that stand out in the courts' duty to children under the Children Act 1989. Note down what you consider the terms 'paramount' and 'welfare' to mean.

Now read below for further information.

'Paramount' means more than the child being the first of a list of considerations by the court. In *J v C* [1970], the court held that 'paramount' means:

> More than placing the child's welfare first. It connotes a process where the course to be followed will be that which is most in the interests of the child's welfare.

It is the only consideration of the court and the duty to consider the welfare of the child will be reflected in the court's decision.

'Welfare' is not statutorily defined by the Children Act 1989 and the court is able to exercise its discretion in each case. It is not uncommon for the court to speak of acting in the best interests of the child. The Court of Appeal will only overrule a decision on the welfare principle where it considers it to be plainly wrong (*G v G (Minors: Custody Appeal)* [1985]).

Scenario 7.5

The welfare principle

In *Re W (A Minor) (Residence Order)* [1992], a couple agreed before their child was born that she would live with her father. Two days after the birth a parental responsibility agreement gave the father parental rights, but the mother then

---

Scenario 7.5 continued

changed her mind and applied for the return of the child. When the judge declined to move the baby pending a welfare officer's report and final determination of the case, the mother appealed. The Court of Appeal held that, although there was no presumption that any child of any age was better off with one parent than the other, it was a rebuttable fact that a tiny baby's interests were best served by being with its mother. The judge was plainly wrong to leave the question of the child's placement until the final hearing, as the child was less than a month old and her welfare required that she should be with her mother.

In child protection proceedings the court must consider a checklist of factors to help it determine what would be in the best interests of the child's welfare (Children Act 1989, section 1(4)). The checklist encourages the court to consider all factors in a holistic way and can help people with a child protection role, such as nurses, to focus on the relevant issues.

Activity 7.4

Coming to a decision on welfare

You have already written what the term 'welfare' means. Imagine that you have been asked to decide on the best interests of a child's welfare. In a group discuss what factors you would take into account in making such a decision. For example, will you allow the child to express his or her wishes?

Now read below for further information.

The welfare checklist requires the court to have regard to the following.

- **The ascertainable wishes and feelings of the child.**
  These will be considered in the light of the child's age and understanding (*Gillick v West Norfolk and Wisbech AHA* [1986]). Unless the child can show sufficient maturity and understanding to exercise a wise choice on the issues, the court will appoint a Children's Guardian, an independent officer of the Children and Family Court Advisory and Support Service experienced in working with children and families, to represent the interests of the child (*Re S (A Minor) (Representation)* [1993]).
- **The child's physical, emotional and educational needs.**
  The court is required to take a wide-ranging view of the needs of the child that goes beyond material and monetary needs. As Lord Justice Griffiths (at 637) stated in *Re P (Adoption: Parental Agreement)* [1985], *Anyone with experience of life knows that affluence and happiness are not necessarily synonymous.*
- **The likely effect of any change in circumstances.**
  The court must consider the impact of change on the child and is encouraged to avoid unnecessary disruption to the life of the child. In *Re B (Minors) (Residence Order)* [1992], the mother of four children left the family home leaving them with their father. She later returned and removed one of the children. The Court of Appeal held that an order for the return of the child to his father and siblings could be made in order to minimise the effect of a change of circumstances on the child.

- **The age, sex, background and any characteristics of the child that the court considers relevant.**
  The age and sex of the child will not conclusively determine the welfare of the child but can be influential. In *Re S (A Minor) (Custody)* [1991], a mother was granted custody of a child, even though she had previously assaulted the child, then disappeared for several weeks leaving the very young child with its father. The Court of Appeal held that there was no presumption that one parent was to be preferred over the other for the purposes of looking after a child. Although it might be expected that young children, especially girls, would remain with their mothers, where there was a dispute over custody this was merely a consideration rather than a presumption.
- **The harm suffered or that a child is at risk of suffering.**
  In *Re G (Children) (Same Sex Partner)* [2006], the court refused to allow a woman and her two children to relocate from the Midlands to Cornwall when her relationship with her same sex partner broke down. The court held that, in the case of a same sex relationship where the care of the children was shared, the children would not distinguish between one woman and another on the grounds of a biological relationship. Therefore, it was necessary for the court in making its determination on the welfare of the children to balance the harm to the children of not allowing the move against the future harm to the children if they were not able to have the relationship with the estranged partner that they needed for their welfare.
- **How capable each parent, and any other person is of meeting the child's needs.**
  In *Humberside County Council v B* [1993], the Court of Appeal held that a court had been wrong to issue an interim care order against the parents who both suffered from schizophrenia. The Court concluded that the magistrates had failed to consider the capability of the parents when determining the welfare of the child.
- **The range of powers available to the court under this Act.**
  This provision requires the court to consider how best to provide for the child's welfare. It is not confined to considering the order requested by the local authority and can instead substitute a different order or no order at all. In *Re O (A Child) (Supervision Order: Future Harm)* [2001], the court substituted a supervision order in place of the care order sought by the local authority as, on the evidence, what was required to protect the child was support and a watching brief on the family, where the mother suffered from recurring episodes of mental health problems that might result in future risk of harm to the child.

Courts must clearly demonstrate that they have considered each element of the welfare checklist when making a decision about the welfare of the child.

Keeping the family together

The Children Act 1989 has a presumption that a child is best looked after within a family where both parents play an equal part. Where difficulties occur, families should be supported to carry out that role unless it is clearly against the best interests of the welfare of the child. Before the introduction of the Children Act 1989, social services departments were seen as needlessly adversarial and the removal of children from the family was the main solution to problems within the family.

Now a range of family support mechanisms and the involvement of other family members are used to provide a nurturing and protective environment for children. In the first five years of the Children Act 1989 there were some 20,000 fewer children in the care system.

Children in need

To encourage work with families, local authorities have a duty to promote the welfare of a child in need by providing appropriate services (Children Act 1989, section 17). The aim is to promote the upbringing of such children by their families.

Activity 7.5

A child in need

In a group, discuss what you consider the meaning of a child in need to be. Write down key points that will indicate that a child is in need. Please do not read the text below until you have completed this exercise.

Now read below for further information.

A child in need is one that:

Is unlikely to achieve or maintain a reasonable standard of health or development without the provision of services by a local authority or their health or development is likely to be significantly impaired or further impaired without the provision of services by a local authority or they are disabled.

(Children Act 1989, section 17(10))

The definition includes children at risk of abuse but can also include other children. For example, a child who is disabled may meet the definition of a child in need but is not necessarily at risk of abuse. The duty to children in need is key to preventative work with particularly vulnerable children and nurses are ideally placed to help identify children who would benefit from intervention by the local authority. Good practice requires the local authority to assess need in an open way that involves the child and their carers, and families have a right to receive sympathetic support and sensitive intervention in their lives (DH, 1997).

The non-intervention principle

The Children Act 1989, section 1(5), provides that a court shall not make an order unless it considers that doing so would be better for the child than making no order at all. The non-intervention or no order principle is one of the most innovative principles of the Act (Bainham, 1990). It requires the court to be satisfied that any order it issues will make a positive contribution to the welfare of the child. This helps avoid unnecessary state intervention and preserves the integrity and independence of the family. As Justice Wall stated in *Re DH (A Minor) (Child Abuse)* [1994]:

Parents should be free wherever possible to bring up their children without interference from courts or other statutory body.

(at 707)

Where nurses are involved in child protection proceedings, they must take note of the no order principle and the initial presumption of the court that no order will be issued. It will be for the agencies involved to rebut this presumption by demonstrating that the grounds for an order are met and that such an order is necessary to promote the welfare of the child.

Avoidance of delay

Delays in child care cases are considered detrimental to the child concerned. Children require stability and prolonged litigation is damaging. Under the Act, courts may be accessed according to the degree of complexity of the case. In applications for care and supervision orders, courts are required to draw up a timetable for disposal of the case. There is a presumption that a full hearing will take place in 12 weeks. The Court of Appeal held in B v B (Minors) (Residence and Care Disputes) [1994] that practitioners had a duty to avoid delay in child cases. Where nurses are asked to provide reports or statements as proof of evidence they must do so without unnecessary delay.

Unified laws and procedures

The Children Act 1989 unifies the laws and procedures relating to the welfare of children. Previously there existed distinct private and public law systems. Now there exists one set of laws that includes provision for both private law matters, where there are disputes within families that cannot be resolved without recourse to the law, and public law matters, which allow for the protection of children suffering significant harm.

The Act introduced a three-tier court system in which cases could be moved according to complexity in order to avoid delay.

Magistrates' courts

Children Act cases are heard by the Family Proceedings Court. The bench is drawn from magistrates on the criminal bench and from the youth court. All applications for care or supervision orders under the Children Act 1989 start in the Family Proceedings Court.

County courts

County courts deal with a wide variety of civil cases, including family proceedings. Cases are normally heard by a judge, and some 50 county courts are designated care centres where specially nominated care judges hear care order applications transferred from the magistrates' courts. A number of county courts are family hearing centres, which deal with contested private law hearings, such as with whom a child should live, and adoption applications, while divorce county courts are able to hear applications relating to children arising out of divorce proceedings.

Any county court may make orders under the Children Act 1989 in the course of other family proceedings, such as when orders need to be made regarding children following an application by a parent for a non-molestation order under the Family Law Act 1996.

The High Court's civil jurisdiction

The Family Division of the High Court hears family proceedings, including Children Act and adoption cases, and appeals from the Family Proceedings Court. Where urgent cases need to be considered, the Court operates a service out of court hours and there is always a High Court judge on call.

Scenario 7.6

Need for an urgent judgment

In Re M (A Minor)(Medical Treatment) [1997], Justice Johnson was on call on a Friday evening when the duty clerk informed him of an application for leave to give a 15-year-old girl a heart transplant against her wishes. With the assistance of the official solicitor, his Lordship was able to gather the necessary evidence and make a ruling in the early hours of Saturday morning. Where there is great urgency, decisions can be made quickly outside normal court hours.

The aim of the five principles of the Children Act 1989 is to ensure that matters of concern regarding children are managed sensitively and with appropriate speed for the benefit of the welfare of the child. This, suggests Dame Butler-Sloss (2003), ensures that the child is viewed by the law and practitioners as a person, not an object of concern.

Significant harm

Prior to the Children Act 1989, there were some 17 routes into care. The welfare principle alone is not robust enough to act as the threshold for state intervention in family life. The minimum requirement that has to be fulfilled before state intervention in a family's life is the risk of significant harm to the child.

Activity 7.6

Significant harm

In a group, discuss what factors you would take into account when determining if a child is suffering or is likely to suffer significant harm. Remember to look at factors that may cause significant harm now and factors that could cause significant harm in the future. Separate your list into present harm and future harm. Some factors may be present in both lists.

Now read below for further information.

Significant harm is the threshold criterion below which state intervention with families cannot be justified. That is, the child is suffering or likely to suffer significant harm (Children Act 1989, section 31(2)).

The phrase is expressed in the present and the future tense. The present tense refers to harm suffered at the time immediately preceding intervention by the child protection authorities.

Scenario 7.7

Applying the threshold criterion

In *Re M (A Minor) (Care Order: Threshold Conditions)* [1994], a court held that the significant harm criterion no longer applied after a father killed the mother of the child who was now being looked after by an aunt. The father was serving life in prison and was therefore no longer a risk to the child.

In *Northamptonshire County Council v S* [1993], the court held that the significant harm criterion still applied even though the children had been removed from their abusive parents and put in the care of their grandparents, as the grandparents had no legal authority over the children and so their parents could remove them at any time. Only where there have been significant changes in circumstances can the court ignore the original circumstances in which action was taken by the child protection authorities.

The future tense element of the threshold criterion relies on speculation about the likelihood of harm. That is, there must be a real possibility of harm to the child.

It need not be proved that the child is more likely to be harmed than not. The standard of proof is the normal civil standard based on the balance of probabilities, not the criminal standard requiring evidence beyond reasonable doubt (*Re H (Minors) (Sexual Abuse: Standard of Proof)* [1996]). However, the House of Lords states that the more serious the allegation the less likely it is to have happened and the more sceptical the courts should be of evidence to prove it. More evidence is required by the courts to prove more serious allegations.

It is not necessary to establish who caused harm to the child. If the harm is attributable to a third party it will only be actionable in care or supervision proceedings if it could reasonably have been prevented by the parent.

Scenario 7.8

Preventable harm

In *Lancashire County Council v W (A Child) (Care Orders: Significant Harm)* [2000], it could not be established whether the parents or a childminder caused injuries to the child. The court held that it did not matter whether it was the parents or the childminder as the childminder was under the supervision and control of the parents.

To satisfy the threshold criterion for state intervention the harm must be significant. This definition incorporates physical and emotional harm and neglect. For example, in *Re O (A Minor) (Care Order: Education Procedure)* [1992], the court held that truanting amounted to harm that could be significant. Minor shortcomings in healthcare or minor deficits in physical, psychological or social development should not require compulsory intervention unless cumulatively they are having, or are likely to have, serious and lasting effects upon the child (DH, 1997). Where the harm relates to health or development, the child is compared with a similar child (Children Act 1989, section 31(10)). The need to use a standard appropriate to the child in question arises because some children have characteristics or developmental difficulties that mean they cannot be expected to be as healthy or well developed as others.

To meet the threshold criterion, the Children Act 1989 requires that the significant harm is attributable either to unreasonable care or to the child being beyond parental control.

Care refers to the physical and emotional support that a reasonable parent would give to the particular child having regard to their needs (*Re B (A Minor) (Care Order: Criteria)* [1993]). Where the child is beyond parental control the fault or innocence of the parents is irrelevant (*Re O (A Minor) (Care Order: Education Procedure)* [1992]).

Powers to safeguard children

Urgent intervention

The need for timely intervention is crucial to the proper protection of children at risk of significant harm.

Scenario 7.9

Failure to act

In *Z v United Kingdom* [2001], Z and his three siblings had been subjected to severe long-term neglect and abuse contrary to the European Convention on Human Rights 1950 (article 3), which granted freedom from torture or inhuman or degrading treatment. The behaviour of the family had been reported to the social services on several occasions, yet they had only acted five years after the first complaint, when the children were placed in emergency care at the insistence of their mother. The court held that the system had failed to protect Z and his siblings, as the state had clearly failed in its obligation to protect the children from ill-treatment of which it had, or ought to have had, knowledge.

Activity 7.7

Protecting children

Before you move on to the next part of this chapter, discuss in a group what actions can be taken and by whom in the following situations:

- a child is being abused and is in need of urgent intervention;
- a mother walked on to a ward and took her sick child away despite being told that the child was severely ill.

Now read below for further information.

Emergency protection orders

Protection for children in urgent need of intervention is provided by an emergency protection order under the Children Act 1989, section 44. The order is intended for use in an emergency rather than as a routine response to concerns about a child or a measure to coerce parents to cooperate with the local authority.

A court may make the order to any person where it is satisfied that there is reasonable cause to believe that the child is likely to suffer significant harm if they are not removed to accommodation provided by the applicant or if they remain where they are being accommodated. The applicant must convince the court of the urgency of the situation. Proof that a child has suffered significant harm in the past will not satisfy the grounds for the order. Emergency protection must be needed in the current circumstances the child faces, not past dangers.

A court may also grant an emergency protection order in cases where enquiries by the local authority or an authorised person (an officer of the National Society for the Prevention of Cruelty to Children (NSPCC)) are being unreasonably frustrated and they are unable to establish if the child is at risk of significant harm and need access to the child as a matter of urgency.

Effect of an emergency protection order

An emergency protection order operates as a direction to comply with a request to produce the child and can include a provision requiring a person to disclose information about the whereabouts of the child (Children Act 1989, section 48). It may authorise the applicant to enter and search for the child named in the order. Should another child be found on the premises, the order will apply to them as well. It is an offence to obstruct the execution of an order.

The emergency protection order authorises the removal of the child or prevents the child's removal from any hospital or other place. It allows the applicant to see the child and if necessary remove them from the home. The court may order that a doctor or a registered nurse accompany the applicant. If the child is produced unharmed, with no likelihood of significant harm, they should not be removed.

If the child is removed, parental responsibility is conferred on the applicant for the duration of the order. The order can last for up to eight days and can be renewed for up to a further seven days. Contact by those with parental responsibility cannot be prevented unless specifically directed in the order. There is no right of appeal against the order but the parents can apply to have it discharged after the initial 72-hour period has elapsed.

As an alternative to removing the child, a court may include an exclusion requirement in an emergency protection order. This allows a perpetrator to be removed from the home instead of the child. To grant the order the court must be satisfied that there is reasonable cause to believe that, if the person is excluded, the child will cease to suffer significant harm or enquiries will cease to be frustrated. There must be another person living in the home who is both able and willing to give the child the care he or she requires.

Police protection

In *X v Liverpool City Council & the Chief Constable of Merseyside Police* [2005], the court held that the removal of children from their family in an emergency should usually be carried out by means of an emergency protection order, as it requires a magistrate to scrutinise the evidence for action before granting an order.

Where such an order is not practical, a police officer may use their powers under the Children Act 1989, section 46. Where a constable has reasonable cause to believe that a child would be likely to suffer significant harm, they may remove the child to suitable accommodation or prevent the child's removal from any hospital, or other place, in which they are being accommodated. The power allows police officers to take immediate action without the need for a court order. A child made subject to the power cannot be kept in police protection for more than 72 hours and no parental responsibility is conferred on the police. A constable using the power must inform the local authority of the steps that have been taken and the reasons for them. If the child is capable of understanding, he or she must also be informed and the officer must take steps to discover the wishes and feelings of the child. As soon as is practicable, the constable will contact the child's parents and inform them of the use of the order and what further steps may be taken with respect to the child. Every police force has an officer designated to enquire further into cases where the police power has been used. Once that officer has completed their enquiries, the child should be released from police protection unless there is evidence to suggest a continued risk of significant harm. The 72-hour period is considered sufficient time to decide what further action needs to be taken to protect the child from significant harm. The designated officer may allow parents contact with a child in police protection if they consider it to be in the child's best interests to do so.

Duty to investigate

The use of an emergency protection order or police power begins a process of continued investigation and assessment of the child's welfare. A local authority has a duty to make such enquiries as they consider necessary to enable them to decide whether to take further action to protect a child from harm or promote the welfare of a child (Children Act 1989, section 47). This duty arises when they are informed that a child in their area is the subject of an emergency protection order or police protection.

The local authority must also investigate when they have reasonable cause to suspect that a child is at risk of significant harm. A local authority must treat as serious any allegations of abuse raised with them by nurses or teachers. In *Re E (Children) (Care Proceedings: Social Work Practice)* [2000], a local authority applied for care orders in respect of three children who had been physically ill treated and showed signs of emotional disturbance. Social services had originally supported the children, but despite warnings from teachers and without proper consideration of the file, had decided to take no further action because of the parents' failure to cooperate. The case had been reopened after another referral from a concerned school and an emergency protection order was made in respect of two of the children and care proceedings were commenced in respect of all the children. It was clear to the court that the children had been left to suffer in totally inadequate conditions for many years. They recommended that every case file should have, at the top or on the front, a chronology recording every significant event. Lack of parental cooperation should never be a reason to close a case, but should inspire closer investigation of the case. The court also stressed that nurses, health visitors and teachers were important sources of information and any referrals by them must be treated with utmost seriousness.

The need to ensure effective interagency working to protect children has now been placed on a statutory footing with the introduction of the Children Act 2004.

Children Act 2004

The aim of the government's strategy for reforming children's services (DH, 2003d) is to ensure that children have the support they need to:

- be safe;
- stay safe;
- enjoy and achieve through learning;
- make a positive contribution to society;
- achieve economic well-being.

The Children Act 2004 provides the legal framework for this reform and it acknowledges that children can only be properly safeguarded if key agencies work together effectively.

Local Safeguarding Children Boards (LSCBs) now oversee the way agencies work together to safeguard and promote the welfare of children (Children Act 2004, section 31).

The investigation of allegations of abuse and subsequent intervention with the child and their family are now conducted in accordance with the policies and procedures established by the LSCBs (HM Government, 2006).

The Children Act 1989 places a duty on health, education and other services to help the local authority to carry out its enquiries under the Children Act 1989, section 47. Professionals, including nurses, who participate in these enquiries are assisted in fulfilling their roles by guidance set out in *Working Together to Safeguard Children* (HM Government, 2006).

Enquiries should always be carried out in such a way as to minimise distress to the child, and to ensure that families are treated sensitively and with respect. This includes the need to explain the purpose and outcome of the enquiries to the parents and child, and being prepared to answer questions openly where this would not affect the safety and welfare of the child (HM Government, 2006).

In the great majority of cases, children remain with their families following an enquiry into an allegation of abuse even though concerns about abuse or neglect have been substantiated. By encouraging cooperation and respect between agencies and families under investigation, it is hoped that constructive working relationships with families will be developed.

Where families refuse to cooperate with the assessment of a child, a child assessment order under the provisions of the Children Act 1989, section 43, may be sought.

Child assessment orders

A child assessment order may be sought where a child's health, development or treatment is a cause for real concern, but where the child is not regarded by the local authority to be in need of urgent intervention. The order is used where repeated attempts to examine and assess the child have failed. Before granting the order the court must be satisfied that there is reasonable cause to suspect that the child is at risk of significant harm, and that an assessment to determine this is unlikely to be made without the order (Children Act 1989, section 43(1)). When granting the order the court will state the date on which the assessment will commence and the order will expire seven days from that date. The effect of the order is to require the child to be produced for assessment. Where a child is of sufficient understanding to make an informed decision, they may refuse to submit to a medical or psychiatric examination or other assessment. Where a nurse is involved in an assessment under this order it will be essential for them to record the consent or refusal of the child to submit to the assessment process.

A child subject to an assessment order may only be kept away from home if it is necessary for the purposes of the assessment and only for the period specified in the order. The child cannot be kept away from home for the convenience of those operating the assessment.

Once the assessment is completed the local authority will decide how to proceed following discussions with those who have been significantly involved in the enquiries and this includes the child and the parents.

Where it is judged that a child may continue to be at risk of suffering significant harm, a child protection conference will be convened (HM Government, 2006).

The aim of this conference is to enable those professionals most involved with the child and family, and the family themselves, to assess all relevant information and plan how best to safeguard and promote the welfare of the child.

The initial child protection conference is responsible for agreeing an outline child protection plan (HM Government, 2006) aimed at:

- ensuring the child is safe and preventing them from suffering further harm;
- promoting the child's health and development;
- supporting the family and wider family members to safeguard and promote the welfare of the child.

Where there is concern that a child continues to suffer or is at risk of suffering significant harm, the local authority (or NSPCC) may apply to the court for a care or supervision order (Children Act 1989, section 31).

Care or supervision orders

Care or supervision orders are the only route into care and there is no way to avoid these proceedings. The courts cannot use their wardship jurisdiction to compel local authorities to look after children (Children Act 1989, section 100). Similarly, a residence order that settles where a child should live cannot be granted in favour of a local authority (Children Act 1989, section 9(2)).

A court cannot make a care order on its own motion. It has no power to force a local authority to take a child into care (Re K [1995]).

A court may make a care or supervision order if:

- the child is, or is likely to, suffer significant harm; and
- the harm is attributable either to unreasonable care (present or potential) or to the child being beyond parental control.

Once the court has established that the threshold criterion has been satisfied, it is able to make a care or supervision order under the Children Act 1989, section 31, if it is in the best interests of the child's welfare to do so.

To reach a decision about the welfare of the child, the court will scrutinise any plan that the local authority has for the care of the child should the order be granted. This must include plans for continued contact with the child's parents, unless the application for the order specifically requests that all contact should be curtailed (Re T (1994)).

Once the order is made, the court hands over the care of the child to the local authority and it no longer has supervision over the local authority's exercise of the care order (S (Children) (Care Order: Implementation of Care Plan) [2002]).

In care and supervision proceedings, the court is being asked to make a long-term order for the protection of the child. The effects of the two orders are different, even though the grounds for granting them are the same. The choice of order depends on the amount of intervention needed to ensure the safety of the child.

A supervision order

Under this order a child would be placed under the supervision of the local authority or a probation officer. That person's duty would be to befriend, advise, assist and supervise the child. Parental responsibility is not granted to the local authority and the child cannot be removed from the family home. The court can impose a wide range of health-related requirements in a supervision order that authorise medical examination and assessment and, in some cases, treatment for the child. A supervision order initially runs for a year and may be extended up to a maximum of three years (Children Act 1989, section 35(1) and part 1 of schedule 3).

A care order

Under a care order a local authority receives a child into its care and takes control of their life. The authority gains parental responsibility for the child and, although parents do not lose their parental responsibility, the local authority can control how they exercise it in relation to their child (Children Act 1989, section 33 (2)).

Once the order is made, the local authority controls the care of the child absolutely, free from court scrutiny. The care order will be carried out in accordance with the care plan agreed by the court and, where necessary, this can include removing the child from the family home immediately or at a later date, where a lack of cooperation or continued risk of significant harm makes this necessary. A care order, which generally cannot be made in respect of a child over 17, or 16 if married, is usually in force until the child is 18 or a court grants an application to have it removed.

Care orders provide for longer-term intervention in a child's life, in order to promote the child's welfare and protect the child from significant harm.

- The United Nations Convention on the Rights of the Child requires the government to have regard to the full spectrum of human rights for all children and to consider children in legislative and policy decisions.
- The Convention says that children have the right to be protected from abuse and the UK provides this protection through the Children Act 1989.
- Nurses have a key role in the identification of children who may have been abused or who are at risk of abuse.
- In the UK, available figures show that there are 32,100 children on child protection registers as being at risk of abuse.
- The Children Act 1989 enshrines the five key principles of holding the child's welfare as paramount; keeping the family together; only intervening where it would make a significant contribution to the welfare of the child; avoiding delay; and unifying laws and procedures.
- The minimum requirement that has to be fulfilled before state intervention in a family's life is the risk of significant harm to the child.
- Protection for children in urgent need of intervention is provided by an emergency protection order under the Children Act 1989.
- A constable who believes a child is suffering significant harm may remove them to suitable accommodation or prevent their removal from hospital, or another place.
- A local authority has a duty to make enquiries to enable them to decide whether to take further action to protect a child from harm or promote the welfare of a child.
- In reforming children's services, the government aims to ensure that children are able to be safe, stay safe, enjoy and achieve through learning, make a positive contribution to society and achieve economic well-being.
- A child assessment order may be sought where a child's health, development or treatment is a cause for real concern, but where the child is not regarded by the local authority to be in need of urgent intervention.
- Care or supervision orders are the only route into care and there is no way for a local authority to avoid these proceedings.
- A supervision order places a child or family member under the supervision of the local authority or a probation officer.
- With a care order a local authority receives a child into its care and takes control of their life by gaining parental responsibility for the child and by controlling how parents exercise their own parental responsibility in relation to the child.

Knowledge review

Now that you've worked through the chapter, how would you rate your knowledge of the following topics?

	Good	Adequate	Poor
1. The five principles of the Children Act 1989.			
2. The concept of significant harm.			
3. The role of the nurse in protecting children.			
4. The powers available to safeguard children from abuse.			

Where you're not confident in your knowledge of a topic, what will you do next?

Further reading

Cobley, C (1995) *Child Abuse and the Law*. London: Cavendish.

Department of Health (DH) (1997) *Children Act 1989: Guidance and regulations*. London: HMSO.

Department of Health (DH) (2003) *Every Child Matters* (Cm 5860). London: The Stationery Office.

Useful websites

www.dfes.gov.uk/publications/childrenactreport The Children Act 1998 Report 2004 and 2005.

www.everychildmatters.gov.uk/strategy/guidance As well as *Every Child Matters*, the website contains information and several other useful documents.

www.nspcc.org.uk Child protection register statistics.

www.opsi.gov.uk/acts/acts1989 Children Act 1989.

www.unicef.org/crc United Nations International Children's Emergency Fund (UNICEF) Conventions on the rights of the child.

Chapter 8

Negligence

NMC Standards of Proficiency

This chapter will address the following NMC *Standards of Proficiency* and *Outcomes to be achieved for entry to the branch programme.*

Manage oneself, one's practice, and that of others, in accordance with *The NMC Code of Professional Conduct: Standards for conduct, performance and ethics*, recognising one's own abilities and limitations.

Outcomes to be achieved for entry to the branch programme:
Demonstrate an awareness of The NMC Code of Professional Conduct: Standards for conduct, performance and ethics:

- commit to the principle that the primary purpose of the registered nurse is to protect and serve society;
- accept responsibility for one's own actions and decisions.

Chapter aims

By the end of this chapter you will be able to:

- explain the tort of negligence;
- describe the elements of a negligence action;
- outline the extent of a nurse's duty of care;
- identify situations where carelessness becomes a crime.

Introduction

Nurses in the course of their duties can make careless mistakes that result in harm to patients in their care. Such mistakes might not be intentional, but the resulting harm can have a profound effect on the life of the patient. To discourage such carelessness and to provide a remedy for those harmed by the mistakes of others, the law imposes a standard of care on nurses that requires them to be careful when caring for patients.

Failing to meet that standard and harming a patient means that the nurse will be accountable for carelessness through the law of negligence.

Claims for compensation as a result of negligence within the NHS have been increasing steadily and are now having an impact on financial resources, as they have a potential value of some £5 billion. In 2006–7, 5,426 claims of clinical negligence and 3,293 claims of non-clinical negligence against NHS bodies were received by the National Health Service Litigation Authority (NHSLA). About £579.3 million was paid out in connection with clinical negligence claims in 2006–7. The NHSLA estimates that the total cost is some £9.09 billion for clinical claims and £0.13 billion for non-clinical claims (NHSLA, 2007).

For the nurse concerned it is undoubtedly a frightening prospect to face a negligence claim. As well as any damages that may be awarded, the nurse faces having their professional integrity and good name challenged in court and the prospect of further action being taken against them by their employer and regulatory body.

Negligence

Where a nurse acts in a careless way and causes an injury to another person, such as a patient, that careless nurse will be liable in negligence for any resulting harm.

Negligence may be defined as an omission to do something a reasonable man [sic] would do or to do something a prudent and reasonable man would not do (*Blyth v Birmingham Waterworks* (1856)).

Scenario 8.1

A nurse's carelessness

In *Bayliss v Blagg and Another* (1954), a nurse failed to heed the concerns of the father of a patient whose leg she had put in plaster. The court found that, although the plaster had been put on with care and skill, there had subsequently been a high degree of carelessness, covering a protracted period of time, where the nurse failed to check for herself or heed the warnings she received of deterioration in the patient's condition. As a result the patient suffered an infection that ate away most of his calf muscle. The court found the nurse negligent and awarded damages to the patient.

A person can claim for damages as a result of loss or harm they have suffered following a nurse's carelessness. Negligence is therefore best defined as actionable harm. If your act or omission causes harm, you could be liable for the civil wrong – known in law as a tort – of negligence. If no harm occurs as a result of the negligent act, a patient cannot bring an action against the nurse.

Activity 8.1

The scope of accountability in nursing

Imagine you have administered the wrong drug to a patient in your care. Fortunately, no harm was done.

- Can you still be held accountable for your actions?
- Who can hold you to account and why?
- What sanctions can be imposed on you?

When answering this question, consider the four spheres of accountability discussed in Chapter 2 (see page 35).

An outline answer is given at the end of the chapter.

Negligence as a tort has been developed in English law under the common law provisions. These are a series of judicial decisions and precedents that have the authority of tests that need to be satisfied if a case is to be successful. A tort is derived from the Norman French word meaning 'wrong' and is now legally defined as a civil wrong. If a member of the public, such as a patient, feels that a tort has been committed against them, they might seek redress from the court. In order to establish negligence in law, three conditions must be met:

- the person who is considered at fault for the negligence, such as the nurse, must owe the patient a duty of care;
- that duty of care must have been breached; this means that the nurse responsible fell below the standard of care expected of them;
- as a result of that breach in the standard of care, harm was caused to the patient.

All three conditions must be satisfied in order to establish liability in the law of negligence.

Duty of care

The first condition to be satisfied in a case of negligence is whether there is a duty of care owed to the individual patient. The tort of negligence does not impose a general duty to act carefully towards everyone. Instead, it lays down standards for particular circumstances and, if someone fails to reach those standards and damage is caused, that is negligence.

These situations are called 'duty situations' and the nature of the relationship gives rise to a duty of care. The courts have also described this duty as a duty to take care or a duty to be careful (*Bolitho v City and Hackney HA* [1998]). That is, there is a legal obligation to ensure that your acts or omissions do not cause harm to the person to whom you owe the duty.

The courts usually rely on previous cases – precedents – to guide them as to when a duty of care arises, and it is well established that the relationship between a health professional and a patient is one that gives rise to a duty of care (*Kent v Griffiths and Others* [2000]).

Your duty of care to the patient arises once you undertake the care and treatment of the patient and therefore assume responsibility for the acts and omissions that make up the nursing interventions you provide (Nathan, 1957).

In novel situations where there is no previous case to follow and it is less clear about whether a duty of care is owed, the court has established a three-stage test.

In *Caparo Industries Plc v Dickman* [1992], the House of Lords provided guidance for establishing a duty of care in novel circumstances. The court held that a duty of care will arise if the following criteria are satisfied.

- **It was reasonably foreseeable that someone would be harmed by a careless act or omission.**
  The test is based on the reasonable foreseeability of harm. That is, would a reasonable person have foreseen that harm would have been caused by the act or omission in question? For example, in *Roe v Ministry of Health* [1954], a man was paralysed when a local anaesthetic was contaminated by a strong disinfectant due to microscopic cracks in the ampoule. The court held that the harm was not foreseeable as the situation was new and a reasonable person would not have foreseen it.

- **It is shown that there is a legal proximity between the parties.**
  The need for a close or proximate relationship with the person harmed was established in *Donoghue v Stevenson* [1932], where a woman claimed damages after drinking ginger beer from a bottle that was contaminated by a decomposing snail. The manufacturer argued that, as there was no contract with Mrs Donoghue, who had not bought the drink, there was no duty of care. However, the court held that in law we owe a duty of care to our *neighbours*, whom the court described as:

  > *persons who are so closely and directly affected by my act or omission that I ought reasonably to have them in contemplation as being so affected when I am directing my mind to the acts or omissions in question.*

  That is, there is a relationship that gives rise to a duty of care – in this case between the manufacturer and consumer of a product. It also includes the nurse–patient relationship. Once you undertake the care and treatment of a patient, the relationship gives rise to a duty of care and continues until that relationship ends. For example, a capable adult patient can absolve you of your duty by refusing the treatment you offer to provide.
- **It is just and reasonable to impose a duty of care in these circumstances.**
  There are some circumstances where the courts believe that imposing a duty is not just and reasonable and so no duty of care arises. For example, in *JD v East Berkshire Community Health NHS Trust* [2003], parents who had unfounded allegations of child abuse made against them sued the Trust for damages due to psychiatric harm. The court held that it was not just and reasonable to impose a duty in these circumstances as the nurse's paramount concern was the child, and if the nurse had suspicions they must be able to report it without having to worry about being sued by parents.

Activity 8.2

Who in law is my neighbour?

While on duty on a ward, you accidentally spill some water in the main corridor. The wet floor is not clearly visible. To whom will you owe a duty of care in this situation? Answer this question by focusing on the neighbour principle.

An outline answer is given at the end of the chapter.

All three elements for establishing a duty of care will not always be separately identifiable. They may overlap or include other factors in some cases. They act as a guide to enable the court to decide whether a duty is owed. Similarly, you ought to take into account these factors when deciding whether you are in a duty situation.

Scenario 8.2

A duty of care

In *Kent v Griffiths and Others* [2000], a woman and her newborn baby suffered harm as a result of an ambulance taking some 30 minutes to arrive to take her to hospital instead of the promised 9 minutes. The ambulance service argued that they did not owe the patient a duty of care as they were an emergency service that provided a service to the public, not to individual patients.

Scenario 8.2 continued

The court held that the ambulance service was part of the health service and owed a duty of care to the patient, as it was reasonably foreseeable that harm would be caused if they acted in a careless way. And, as they knew the name and address of the patient, they had a legal proximity in the same way as other health professionals had with their patients and it was, therefore, just and reasonable to impose a duty of care on the ambulance service towards their patients. By taking so long to arrive without reasonable excuse was careless and a breach of that duty of care.

The scope of the duty of care

The scope of the duty of care owed by a nurse to a patient is very wide and covers every facet of your involvement with the patient. Lord Diplock, in *Sidaway v Bethlem Royal Hospital* [1985], described it as a single comprehensive duty covering all the ways in which a nurse is called on to exercise their skill and judgement in the improvement of the physical and mental condition of the patient. The scope of your duty of care has already been found to include:

- the care given to your patients;
- giving advice to your patient or to another about the patient;
- explaining risks inherent in a procedure to patients;
- the standard of your handwriting when giving instructions regarding a patient;
- the standard of your record keeping in terms of legibility and content;
- the timing of a decision to act;
- seeking the assistance of others;
- failing to recognise the limits of your competence;
- failing to report substandard care.

Breach in the standard of care

Once it is established that the defendant owed a duty of care to the claimant, the second question is whether that duty was breached. That is, did the standard of care fall below that required by law?

Generally, the standard of care is based on the 'reasonable man' test. As cited earlier, in *Blyth v Birmingham Waterworks Co* (1856), it was held that negligence is the omission to do something a reasonable man would do or do something a prudent and reasonable man would not do. Both what you do and what you fail to do can be equally culpable when establishing negligence.

Scenario 8.3

Negligence by omission

In *Goorkani v Tayside Health Board* [1991], a doctor was found negligent when he failed to tell a patient of the risk of irreversible infertility at the time of prescribing chlorambucil for Behcet's disease.

The risk of infertility when used over the longer term rose to 95 per cent and this transpired in Mr Goorkani's case.

In *Hall v Brooklands Auto Racing Club* [1933], the characteristics of a reasonable man were described by the court:

> A reasonable man is sometimes described as the man in the street or the man on the Clapham omnibus or . . . the man who takes the magazines at home and in the evening pushes the lawn mower in his shirt sleeves.
>
> (Lord Justice Greer at 244)

Activity 8.3

The reasonable man

What do you think the judge was trying to say about the standard of care generally required at law in his description of the reasonable man?

Now read the following paragraph for the answer.

By describing the reasonable man in this way Lord Justice Greer was emphasising that the standard of care generally expected in law is that of the ordinary or average person in that situation. That is, what would an ordinary person have done in the same circumstances?

For example, a reasonable person would know what adults learn from experience – that rivers are dangerous, that fires burn, etc. They would also take extra care if they knew that a person had a particular sensitivity, such as an allergy, or that a woman was pregnant. The reasonable person would also take greater precautions where the likelihood of harm was serious and would not ignore even a small risk if it could be avoided simply.

Scenario 8.4

The reasonable man and the cricket ball

In *Bolton v Stone* [1951], a woman was struck by a cricket ball when standing on a road some way from a cricket match. The court held that the cricketer had not been negligent, as a reasonable man would not have foreseen that such an exceptional cricket stroke would have not only travelled so far but then gone on to hit a pedestrian on a quiet country road.

However, Lord Reid pointed out that he would have reached a different conclusion if he had thought that the risk had been other than extremely small, because a reasonable man considering the matter of safety would not disregard any risk unless it was extremely small.

Judging the skilled person

Where the person considered to be at fault for a negligent act or omission is a professional, skilled person, the law modifies the reasonable man test to take account of the skill involved. In *Bolam v Friern HMC* [1957], the court established that:

> The test is that of the ordinary skilled person exercising and professing to have that special skill. A professional need not possess the highest expert skill as it is well established in law that it is sufficient if they exercise the ordinary skill of an ordinary competent professional exercising that particular skill or art.

The test is well established in healthcare law and is known as the *Bolam* test. In *Bolitho v City & Hackney HA* [1998], the House of Lords described the *Bolam* test as the *locus classicus* (the traditional basis) of the test for the standard of care required of a doctor or any other person professing some skill or competence.

The test applies to any profession, including the nursing profession, and it was made clear in *Gold v Haringey HA* [1987] that:

> No matter what profession it may be, the common law does not impose on those who practise it any liability for damage resulting from what in the result turned out to have been errors of judgment, unless the error was such as no reasonably well-informed and competent member of that profession could have made.

The standard of care will, therefore, be determined by what a responsible body of professional opinion would have done in the same situation. In nursing practice the standard of care will be determined by what a responsible body of nursing opinion would have done in the same situation.

This approach allows for different schools of thought within a profession. As long as the practice conforms to a standard accepted by a responsible body of opinion, it meets the standard required in law.

Scenario 8.5

Is there a best standard?

In *Maynard v West Midlands RHA* [1984], two consultants treating a patient for a chest complaint thought she was suffering from tuberculosis, but also considered that she might be suffering from Hodgkin's disease. Before obtaining the result of a tuberculosis test, they performed an exploratory operation to see if she was suffering from Hodgkin's disease. It showed that she had tuberculosis, but the patient suffered damage to a nerve affecting her vocal cords, which caused a speech impairment – an inherent risk of the operation.

The patient sued, claiming that the consultants had been negligent in deciding to carry out the operation before obtaining the result of the tuberculosis test, which would have taken seven weeks.

Expert medical evidence was called on both sides concerning whether the operation should have been carried out. The judge preferred the patient's expert evidence, which said the consultants should have waited, and awarded damages against the hospital.

On appeal, the House of Lords held that it was not sufficient to show that there was a body of competent opinion, which considered that that a decision was wrong, if there also existed a body of professional opinion, equally competent, which supported the decision as being reasonable in the circumstances.

It had to be recognised that differences of opinion and practice existed in the health professions and therefore, although the court might prefer one body of opinion to the other, it was not a basis for a conclusion that there had been negligence.

The *Bolam* test imposes a higher standard of care on health professionals than is generally required when using the reasonable man test. The law requires a person professing to have a particular skill or art to exercise to the standard of the ordinary professional skilled to that level. Two important qualifications of the standard emerge from this principle.

First, the more a professional puts themselves forward as an expert, the higher is the standard expected of them. It is the post, not the person, that carries the duty. A ward sister is putting herself forward as a person with greater skill than a more junior grade member of the nursing staff. The law expects a higher standard of care from the ward sister than from her junior colleagues.

Scenario 8.6

Higher standard when putting yourself forward as an expert

In *Smith v Brighton and Lewes Hospital Management Committee* [1958], a woman lost her balance due to damage to a cranial nerve caused by receiving four injections of streptomycin above 30 prescribed by the doctor. Junior nurses had given the injections, but it was the ward sister who was held liable for negligence as it was found to be her role, as a person in a position of greater competence and expertise, to ensure that the stop date for the treatment was clearly marked on the medication administration chart.

Second, the requirement to perform to the standard of the ordinary person exercising that skill means that there is a minimum level of competence below which no person can fall. Inexperience is, therefore, no defence to an allegation of negligence. If you profess to have a particular skill, you must perform to the standard of the ordinary nurse.

Scenario 8.7

The standard of the average road user

In *Nettleship v Weston* [1971], a learner driver was given lessons by an instructor who made sure the car was properly insured. Weston was a careful learner, but on the third lesson she failed to straighten out after turning left and struck a lamp standard, breaking Nettleship's kneecap.

The court held that a learner driver owes a duty to their instructor to drive with proper skill and care, the test being that of the ordinary careful driver. It was no defence to say they were a learner doing their best. The duty of care owed by a learner driver was the same as that owed by every driver, and Weston was liable for damages.

An important way of ensuring that you do not carelessly harm a patient by practising beyond your competence is to acknowledge the limitations of your practice and seek more senior assistance. This will ensure that you benefit from the help and advice of that colleague. It will also demonstrate that you have discharged your duty of care towards your patient.

Should any harm now occur, it will be the senior professional who will be held liable for negligence, as they are putting themselves forward as an expert and a higher standard of care is expected of them. For example, in *Wilsher v Essex HA* [1988], a baby was born prematurely and was placed in a special baby care unit. The baby needed oxygen and the junior doctor inserting the catheter to measure blood gases was inexperienced and asked a senior colleague, a senior registrar, to check the catheter. The catheter was wrongly inserted into an umbilical vein instead of an artery and the baby was supersaturated with oxygen. He developed retrolental fibroplasia, which resulted in blindness. The court held that, as the junior doctor had asked a more senior doctor to check his work, he had discharged his duty of care to the senior doctor and could not be liable in negligence.

Activity 8.4

Unsure what to do?

What action would you take if you were unsure of how to carry out a nursing intervention on a patient in your care?

An outline answer is given at the end of the chapter.

Emergencies

One exception to the principle that a nurse will be judged according to the standard of reasonably experienced nurses in their field is provided by emergency treatment.

In relation to treatment decisions taken in an emergency, a nurse will not be found negligent simply because the reasonably competent nurse would have made a different decision, given more time and information.

In *Wilson v Swanson* (1956), the Supreme Court of Canada held that there was no negligence when a health professional had to make an immediate decision whether to treat, when the treatment was subsequently found to have been unnecessary.

Moreover, the standard of skill itself required in the execution of treatment may be somewhat lower. As Lord Justice Mustill commented in *Wilsher v Essex HA* [1988]:

> An emergency may overburden the available resources, and, if an individual is forced by circumstances to do too many things at once, the fact that he does one of them incorrectly should not lightly be taken as negligence.

The role of the courts in determining the standard of care

Generally, the courts are content to allow the profession to set the standard of care for a particular treatment or intervention. The essence of the *Bolam* test is that you act in accordance with a practice accepted by a responsible body of professional opinion.

However, the court is the final arbiter of the professional standard of care and, although it must accept that there are different schools of thought about how to best provide treatment within a profession, it can reject a standard where it does not consider that the standard stands up to logical analysis (*Bolitho v City and Hackney HA* [1998]).

Activity 8.5

Does the evidence stand up to logical analysis?

In *Hucks v Cole* (1968), Mrs Hucks was expecting her third child when she noticed a septic spot on her finger. She gave birth three days later in hospital and the following day a nurse noticed the spot and another one on her toe. The doctor prescribed a five-day course of tetracycline and sent a swab to pathology.

The pathologist's report stated that the bacteria was resistant to tetracycline but the doctor decided to stick to the five-day course he had prescribed.

Activity 8.5 continued

> Hucks was discharged at the end of the five days despite the septic spots not having healed and later developed fulminating septicaemia and was seriously ill.
>
> At the trial, evidence was given by other doctors that they would not have changed the prescribed treatment.
>
> Do you think that the doctor's actions stand up to logical analysis?
>
> Now read below for the answer.

In the *Hucks v Cole* (1968) case, the judge held that, despite the evidence of the doctors, no reasonable doctor would have allowed a patient to continue with a course of treatment when they knew it to be ineffective. The standard of care suggested by the doctors did not stand up to logical analysis and would be rejected.

This was later approved by the House of Lords in *Bolitho v City and Hackney HA* [1998], when they held that:

> [Where], in a rare case, it can be demonstrated that the professional opinion is not capable of withstanding logical analysis, the judge is entitled to hold that the body of opinion is not reasonable or responsible.

(Lord Browne-Wilkinson at 240)

It is essential, therefore, that you base your practice on sound evidence and research. You will not be exonerated because others too are negligent or common professional practice is slack (*Reynolds v North Tyneside HA* [2002]). You must keep your practice up to date and inform your practice by reference to improvements and amendments introduced through changes in the law (see page 38).

Guidance on best practice and standard of care

To improve care standards, NHS Trusts have policies and procedures to inform best practice. These are supplemented by guidance from bodies such as the National Institute for Health and Clinical Excellence (NICE), and professional organisations such as the Royal College of Nursing (RCN). Nurses are able to use these to inform their practice. For example, in *Sutton v Population Services Family Planning Programme* [1981], a nurse was found to be negligent when she failed to follow the correct procedure for referring a patient with a lump in her breast to a doctor.

However, the value of such guidance is only as good as the evidence upon which it is based. If it is not based on sound research, the court may reject it as not standing up to logical analysis.

Scenario 8.8

Logical analysis

In *Reynolds v North Tyneside HA* [2002], a woman who was admitted in labour was not given a vaginal examination for some six hours, at which point a prolapsed cord was discovered and an emergency caesarean was carried out. The child suffered cerebral palsy and sued. The hospital argued that its policy did not require the immediate vaginal examination of the woman; however, the pre-eminent textbook of the day suggested that such an examination was necessary where a woman was in labour.

The court held that the hospital policy was not based on sound research evidence and did not stand up to logical analysis, and that there had been a breach in the standard of care causing harm to the child. The hospital was therefore negligent.

Causation: the breach in the standard of care caused harm

Once it is established that, due to the carelessness of the nurse, the standard of care required in law has been breached, it is necessary to consider what effect this had on the patient. This stage is known as 'causation' or the 'causal link'. It must be established that the breach in the standard of care caused the harm.

It is generally for the person who has suffered the wrong (the claimant) to prove causation. The claimant must prove on the balance of probabilities that care fell below the standard of a reasonably competent person and caused the harm. There is a distinction between causation in fact and causation in law.

Causation in fact is based on the 'but for test'. That is, but for your carelessness the patient would not have suffered harm.

Scenario 8.9

A case of too much arsenic

In *Barnett v Chelsea and Kensington Hospital Management Committee* [1969], a night watchman was taken to a cottage hospital complaining of stomach pain. The doctor had flu and told the nurse to ask the patient to go and see his GP. The patient subsequently died of arsenic poisoning before seeing his GP.

The court decided that the doctor who had refused to see the man had acted irresponsibly, but was not negligent, as the doctor's actions did not contribute to the death of the night watchman. He had ingested so much arsenic that he would have died even if the doctor had seen him.

Causation in law requires the court to determine whether the defendant is liable as a matter of law. This is determined by the principle that the defendant will not be held liable in law if the damage is too remote from the original negligent act. For example, in *French v Chief Constable of Sussex* [2006], a police officer claimed damages for psychiatric harm caused when a fatal shooting occurred during an armed robbery. The officer argued that it was his employer's negligent handling of the robbery that had resulted in the fatal shooting and caused him psychiatric harm. The court rejected his claim, holding that, as he did not witness the shooting, the harm he suffered was too remote from the incident and was not reasonably foreseeable.

Res ipsa loquitur

While it is generally for the complainant to prove that a breach in the standard of care caused them harm, there is a principle that allows the burden of proof to shift in certain circumstances.

The principle of *res ipsa loquitur*, or 'the thing speaks for itself', applies when three key conditions are present. That is:

- there is no explanation for the accident;
- harm does not normally happen if care is taken; and
- the instrument causing the accident is in the defendant's control.

The principle, when it applies, requires the respondent to show that they did not act negligently by shifting the burden of proof from the complainant to the respondent.

Scenario 8.10

Res ipsa loquitur

In *Saunders v Leeds Western HA* [1993], an otherwise healthy four-year-old boy suffered a cardiac arrest and brain damage during a routine arthoplasty operation. The theatre team argued that his heart stopped abruptly without warning; however, expert evidence argued that an otherwise healthy child's heart does not simply stop. The judge held that the principle of *res ipsa loquitur* applied, as there was no reasonable explanation for the incident, expert evidence had shown that harm does not normally happen if care is taken, and the instruments that caused the incident were under the control of the hospital. As the theatre could offer no other explanation for what had occurred, the judge found them negligent.

Negligence as a crime

Negligence is generally associated with the civil law. It is the law's way of imposing a standard of care on professionals such as nurses, and it provides redress by way of compensation for those harmed by another's careless act or omission.

In extreme cases the negligent act of a nurse can cause the death of a patient. The nurse may then be liable to prosecution for manslaughter as a result of their gross negligence. In *R v Bateman* [1925], the court decided that gross negligence occurs when someone shows such disregard for the life and safety of other persons as to constitute a crime worthy of punishment. In healthcare the issue of gross negligence arose in *R v Misra & Srivastava* [2004], where two doctors were found guilty of gross negligence when they failed to heed the warnings of nurses that a patient was seriously ill. The patient subsequently died of toxic shock. The judge held that:

> A health professional would be told that grossly negligent treatment which exposed a patient to the risk of death, and caused it, would constitute manslaughter.

This was the case in *R v Adomako* [1995], where the defendant, an anaesthetist, failed to notice for four minutes that an endotracheal tube had become disconnected during an operation. Although an alarm sounded, the tube was not checked until the patient suffered a cardiac arrest. An expert witness for the prosecution stated that a competent anaesthetist should have spotted the problem within 15 seconds. The House of Lords held that gross negligence would occur where a patient dies as the result of:

- a health professional displaying an indifference to an obvious risk of injury to the patient;

- a health professional being aware of the risk of injury to the patient but deciding to run the risk;
- a health professional's attempt to avoid a known risk was so grossly negligent that it deserves to be punished;
- a health professional displays inattention or a failure to avert a severe risk.

Based on these tests, a nurse could be convicted of manslaughter if the act or omission exposes the patient to the risk of death and subsequently causes the patient's death.

Where a nurse is found guilty of such an offence, they are likely to receive a custodial sentence.

Scenario 8.11

Nurses' gross negligence

Two nurses were convicted of killing an elderly patient at a nursing home through neglect (Sinclair, 2003). The resident died from septicaemia resulting from pressure sores the 'size of a fist' that developed while she was a resident at a nursing home on the Isle of Man.

A jury found the nursing services manager at the home and his deputy guilty of manslaughter due to gross negligence in their care of the resident. They argued that the system, not them, was to blame, but the court found that they were in charge of the patient's care and their grossly negligent failure had caused the patient's death.

Accountability

As a registered nurse, you are not only accountable to the patient through the law of negligence. As shown in Chapter 2, you are also accountable to your employer through contract and to the Nursing and Midwifery Council (NMC) through the Nursing and Midwifery Order 2001. Even if you show that your carelessness did not cause harm, you are likely to face investigation by your employer and the NMC.

Under contract law, your employer will pay any damages for liability in negligence through the principle of vicarious liability. This requires that an employer is liable for the negligent acts or omissions of their employee in the course of their employment. The liability arises whether or not such an act or omission was specifically authorised by the employer.

In return for this protection, employers expect their employees to carry out their duties with due care and skill. They can hold you to account through reasonable disciplinary measures, which could include dismissal, if an investigation reveals misconduct.

Under the terms of your contract of employment, you owe your employer a duty of care and undertake to work with due skill and diligence. If you breach that duty by being negligent, it is open to the employer to sue you for the compensation they have had to pay to a patient (*Lister v Romford Ice and Cold Storage Co Ltd* [1957]).

It is essential, therefore, that you carry indemnity insurance to cover you for any damages for which you are personally liable. Currently, the easiest way of obtaining such insurance is to join a professional organisation such as the RCN or Unison.

The European Union is proposing a directive on safe, high-quality and efficient cross-border healthcare, which includes a requirement that health professionals will require to have indemnity insurance in order to practise (European Commission, 2007).

The NMC has a statutory duty to protect the public and, if they receive a complaint, could investigate your conduct and competence. Although the NMC follows the common law standard of care reflected in the *Bolam* test, they do not require harm to have occurred in order to find you guilty of professional misconduct.

Therefore, even though you may not be found liable in negligence, action could still be taken by your employer and regulatory body.

C H A P T E R   S U M M A R Y

- Although being sued for negligence is a rare event in nursing, increasing litigation is a real trend in healthcare with the current NHS liability bill exceeding £4 billion.
- Where a nurse acts in a careless way and causes an injury to another person, such as a patient, that careless nurse will be liable in negligence for any resulting harm.
- Negligence is best defined as actionable harm.
- In order to establish negligence in law, three conditions must be met: the nurse must owe the patient a duty of care; that duty of care must be breached; and, as a result, harm was caused to the patient.
- The relationship between a nurse and a patient is one that gives rise to a duty of care.
- This duty covers all the ways in which a nurse is called upon to exercise their skill and judgement in the improvement of the physical and mental condition of the patient.
- As a skilled professional you are expected to carry out your duties to the standard of the ordinary skilled person exercising and professing to have that special skill.
- The standard of care is determined by what a responsible body of professional opinion would have done in the same situation.
- The more a nurse puts themselves forward as an expert, the higher the standard expected of them.
- Inexperience is no defence to an allegation of negligence.
- The court can reject a professional standard where it does not consider that the standard stands up to logical analysis.
- The principle of *res ipsa loquitur* applies when there is no explanation for the accident, where harm does not normally happen if care is taken, and where the instrument causing the accident is in the defendant's control.
- Grossly negligent treatment that exposes a patient to the risk of death, and causes it, constitutes manslaughter.
- For registered nurses, liability may extend to other spheres of accountability and may draw sanctions from the employer and the regulatory body.
- It is essential that you carry indemnity insurance to cover you for any damages for which you are personally liable.

Activities: brief outline answers

8.1 *The scope of accountability in nursing (page 145)*

You can still be held to account for your actions as there are four spheres of accountability generally attributed to a registered nurse.

Although the patient cannot sue for negligence as no harm occurred, you are still accountable to:

- society through the public law where you may face criminal prosecution;
- the employer through contract law for misconduct;
- the profession through the Nursing and Midwifery Order 2001 for professional misconduct.

8.2 *Who in law is my neighbour? (page 147)*

The courts have held that in law you owe a duty of care to your neighbours who the court describe as:

- persons who are so closely and directly affected by your act or omission that you ought reasonably to have them in contemplation as being so affected when directing your mind to the acts or omissions in question.

In the case of an accidental spill, you would therefore owe a duty to those persons walking along that corridor because it is reasonably foreseeable that they could be harmed if they slipped on that water.

8.4 *Unsure what to do? (page 152)*

Given the decision in *Wilsher v Essex Health Authority* [1988] you would be well advised to seek the supervision of a more senior colleague. Should any harm now occur, it would be the senior professional who would be held liable for negligence as they have put themselves out as an expert and a higher standard of care would be expected of them.

Knowledge review

Now that you've worked through the chapter, how would you rate your knowledge of the following topics?

	Good	Adequate	Poor
1. The elements of a negligence action.			
2 The standard of care required of you as a skilled professional.			
3 The circumstances in which negligence could become a criminal offence.			

Where you are not confident in your knowledge of a topic, what will you do next?

Further reading

Bolitho v City and Hackney HA [1998] AC 232.

Department of Health (2003) *Making Amends: Clinical negligence reform.* London: The Stationery Office.

Department of Health (2003) *An Organisation with a Memory.* London: Department of Health.

Useful websites

www.bailii.org British and Irish Legal Information Institute.

www.lexisnexis.co.uk LexisNexis is a leading provider of legal information for professionals. An Athens account is required for access.

www.nhsla.com National Health Service Litigation Authority.

www.sweetandmaxwell.co.uk/online/lawtel Sweet and Maxwell are leading publishers of legal information. An Athens account is required for access.

Chapter 9

Record keeping

NMC Standards of Proficiency

This chapter will address the following NMC *Standards of Proficiency* and *Outcomes to be achieved for entry to the branch programme.*

Undertake and document a comprehensive, systematic and accurate nursing assessment of the physical, psychological, social and spiritual needs of patients, clients and communities.

Outcomes to be achieved for entry to the branch programme:
Contribute to the development and documentation of nursing assessments by participating in comprehensive and systematic nursing assessment of the physical, psychological, social and spiritual needs of patients and clients.

Formulate and document a plan of nursing care, where possible, in partnership with patients, clients, their carers and family and friends, within a framework of informed consent.

Outcomes to be achieved for entry to the branch programme:
Contribute to the planning of nursing care, involving patients and clients and, where possible, their carers.

Evaluate and document the outcomes of nursing and other interventions.

Outcomes to be achieved for entry to the branch programme:
Contribute to the evaluation of the appropriateness of nursing care delivered:

- contribute to the documentation of the outcomes of nursing interventions.

Demonstrate sound clinical judgement across a range of differing professional and care delivery contexts.

Outcomes to be achieved for entry to the branch programme:
Recognise situations in which agreed plans of nursing care no longer appear appropriate and refer these to an appropriate accountable practitioner:

- accurately record observations made and communicate these to the relevant members of the health and social care team.

Chapter aims

By the end of this chapter you will be able to:

- define a health record;
- outline the two purposes of a health record;
- describe what must be included in a record entry;
- discuss the elements of good record keeping;
- consider the role of audit in raising the standard of record keeping;
- compare and contrast the right of access to records of patients who are living with access to the records of patients who have died.

Introduction

Record keeping is a crucial aspect of a nurse's duty. It remains an instance where failing in this duty can lead to your name being removed from the professional register.

This chapter considers how you should write records to ensure that the legal requirements are met and, by drawing on case law, it highlights the consequences for nurses of failing to meet those requirements.

Scenario 9.1

Struck off for failing to keep adequate records

A nurse from Coventry was removed from the national register after failing to keep accurate records for patients in her care (NMC, 2002). She was found guilty of seven charges of misconduct. The NMC's Competence and Conduct Committee heard that she failed to ensure that care plans were prepared for several patients covering issues such as diabetes, pain management and dietary needs. On one occasion, she failed to notify staff of a patient's increased risk of haemorrhage following a drug error. The NMC found that the nurse had systematically neglected a basic and crucial duty – to keep proper records for the management of patient care.

What is a health record?

A health record is any electronic or paper information recorded about a person for the purpose of managing their healthcare (Data Protection Act 1998, section 68(1)(a)). Health records include a variety of patient records that are held or filed within a hospital practice, not just the main doctor's record. They include nursing records, health visiting records, X-rays, pathology reports, outpatients' reports, pharmacy records, etc. Together they form a record of the care and treatment a patient has received.

Activity 9.1

Purpose of record keeping

Why do you believe the NMC regards record keeping as such an important nursing duty? Write down what you consider to be the purpose of keeping nursing records.

Now read below for further information.

The purpose of record keeping

The primary purpose of keeping records is to have an account of the care and treatment given to a patient. This allows progress to be monitored and a clinical history to be developed. The clinical record allows for continuity of care by facilitating treatment and support. It is an integral part of care that is every bit as important as the direct care provided to patients.

As well as their clinical function, records have a very important legal purpose. Records provide evidence of your involvement with a patient. Therefore, they need to be sufficiently detailed to demonstrate this involvement.

Scenario 9.2

The legal function of records

In *Saunders v Leeds Western HA* [1993], a fit four-year-old child suffered cardiac arrest and brain damage during an arthoplasty operation. The theatre team argued that the patient's pulse had simply stopped abruptly. This was rejected by the court. As there was no evidence in the records of a sequence of events leading to the pulse stopping the court found the health authority liable in negligence.

Remember that the standard of proof in civil cases is the balance of probability. That is, if the weight of evidence is 51 per cent in your favour the case is won. As a nurse's contact with patients is mainly on a one-to-one basis, records made at the time of, or soon after, seeing a patient often provides the necessary evidence to tip the evidence in your favour. For example, in *McLennan v Newcastle HA* [1992], a patient claimed she had not been told of the relatively high risk associated with her operation. The surgeon, however, had written in the notes at the time that the risks were explained and understood by the patient. This contemporaneous record persuaded the judge that the patient had probably been told about the risks and the case failed.

Legal implications of records

The Data Protection Act 1998 defines a health record very widely. In litigation that definition becomes wider still. The discovery process of a case allows any material document to be used as evidence. Any document that records any aspect of the care of a patient can be required as evidence before a court of law or before any of the regulatory bodies. There is no restriction on access to these documents. The rules of the court demand that all documents are produced (Rules of the Supreme Court Order 24). It is important, therefore, that nurses do not view record keeping as a mechanistic process. What you write does matter. In litigation the outcome is not based on truth but proof. If it is not in the notes it can be difficult to prove it happened. Cases are won and lost on the strength of records. The secret of success in court is preparation, so winning in court could be said to be:

- 96 per cent preparation;
- 2 per cent luck;
- 2 per cent law.

Next time you write in notes, remember that you may be relying on them as evidence in court. They are of little value to you if they do not contain the information necessary to demonstrate that you have discharged your duty of care to the patient with professional skill and diligence. Records are never neutral; they will either support or condemn you.

Activity 9.2

What should be recorded by nurses

Write down the information you feel needs to be included in a patient's nursing record.

Now read below for further information.

What to include

Records need to be sufficiently detailed to show that you have discharged your duty of care. An evidence-based care plan and regular progress reports form the backbone of this detail. To be useful in evidence, however, the record needs to show much more. In *Marriott v West Midlands HA* [1999], a GP was found negligent when he failed to refer back to hospital a man who suffered a head injury in a fall and was still having headaches, lethargy and appetite loss a week later. As this was a home visit, the GP had not taken the man's records with him and was heavily hampered in court by not being able to recount the detail and results of the examination he carried out or why he decided not to refer the patient back to hospital.

It can be seen from *Marriott* that an incomplete or inaccurate record can be fatal to a case. In this instance, details of the examination were missing, but equally damning was the lack of evidence as to why the doctor decided to wait and see. Decisions about care must be included in the patient's record. If you decide that a particular form of treatment or care should be delayed, say so. If you decide to wait and see before you call for a doctor or other assistance, record why you decided to wait.

Decisions about care and treatment are often taken on a multidisciplinary basis. Your records must include the background to the discussion and its outcome. This will indicate the reason for the decision and corroborate the account of other team members. Records must also corroborate any other legal requirement or form completed by the patient in your presence. For example, if a patient signs a consent form, that should be recorded and details discussed should be included. Details of telephone calls made, even if unanswered, to the patient or to others about the patient, and discussions arising from them with date and time, should be included as should referrals to specialist practitioners. Where there are particular concerns, these telephone conversations should be confirmed in a letter.

Scenario 9.3

Victoria Climbié Inquiry

Victoria Climbié died as the result of systematic abuse by her aunt (DH, 2003b). The Inquiry into her death focused on the transfer of the case from a neighbouring social services department. The social worker assigned to her case told the Inquiry that she had contacted the social services department, who told her the family had moved out of the borough, so the case was closed.

Social services denied the conversation took place and the department was still seeing Victoria and her aunt in December 1999 – fully four months after she was referred.

The social worker admitted that she could not remember exactly when the phone conversation had taken place, nor had she dated the entry about the phone call in Victoria's files.

She also had record entries with uneven spaces between them, leading the barrister to the Inquiry to suggest that the note about the phone call to social services was added after the girl's murder in an effort to explain away the fact that she had done nothing with this referral.

Team members occasionally have differences of opinion on patient care. Any expression of dissent you have with another nurse, doctor or pharmacist should be recorded, and included should be the facts leading to the disagreement, the reason why you object and, importantly, what follow-up action was taken.

Views of patients and relatives

A further essential entry must be the views of patients and their relatives. It is useful to differentiate the views of patients and relatives and your own entry by using quotation marks. For example, 'I'm in agony with the pain'. Relatives are an important source of progress or concern about patients. They know the patient well and notice changes in condition more quickly as a result. Their views must be recorded and responded to.

Scenario 9.4

The concerns of relatives must be recorded

In a complaint against *Hastings and Rother NHS Trust* put by *Mrs M and Mrs N* (Health Service Commissioner, 1999), concerning a man who died from an intestinal obstruction, the Health Service Commissioner (the ombudsman) found that the concerns of a patient's relatives were not recorded in the nursing notes. This he found to be a significant oversight. In evidence, the nurses had stated that they would only record conversations with relatives where there was a real concern or anxiety raised.

Q3 DOCUMENTATION
• important issues in relation to record keeping + discuss + relate to care (x 100)
• (written legibly)

Records must be written legibly

It is essential that all records, instructions, prescriptions or referrals for treatment be written legibly and indelibly. Records are the key communication tool between nurses. They allow for continuity of care. It is essential that record entries can be read and this begins with the clarity of the entry. Clarity requires ink that contrasts with the paper being used for entries. For white paper use black ink as this gives the greatest contrast and best clarity when copied. There is a growing trend to use different colour paper for medical, nursing and other entries in shared records. It is essential that the colour chosen facilitates copying. In litigation a record will be copied to each of the relevant parties. That means that, on average, some 20 copies will be made. Records are of little use as evidence if the writing cannot be read due to deterioration in clarity when photocopied.

The standard of your handwriting is also a requirement of your duty of care to a patient. If care is initiated by you through a care plan and harm results because others could not read your writing, liability in negligence is likely to arise.

Scenario 9.5

A doctor with poor handwriting

A good analogy is the case of *Prendergast v Sam and Dee* [1989], in which an illegible prescription resulted in the patient being given the wrong drug and this caused harm. The pharmacist was held to be 75 per cent liable for that harm. For his poor handwriting, the GP was found to be 25 per cent liable. The Court of Appeal held that there is a duty to write clearly so that busy or careless staff can read your instructions.

Legibility extends to the signature of the person who made the entry. Identifying the people and therefore witnesses involved in an incident is crucial to building a successful case. As well as a signature, the name in print or block capitals and grade of the person writing should be noted at least once in the notes during the course of the record. As a useful back-up, the Human Resources Department or GP practice will often hold a signature bank with forwarding addresses, especially if there is a frequent turnover of staff, so that staff who have left can be identified should they be required as a witness to an incident at a later date.

Writing with indelible ink or typeface is essential for two reasons. First, the record must stand the test of time. It may be many years before it is referred to again and a faded record is of little value as evidence. It is usual for several years to pass before an incident goes to court to be decided. Cases generally take three to six years to resolve and can often go on for much longer.

Scenario 9.6

Twenty-one years before a case came to court

In *Reynolds v North Tyneside HA* [2002], a woman argued that she had suffered cerebral palsy as a result of the negligent mismanagement of her mother's labour some 21 years earlier. The patient's records and hospital policy were central to the case. In this instance, the patient's records were in good condition and properly completed. They showed that staff attending the birth had acted according to hospital policy. It was the hospital policy that was found to be incorrect and the court found for the woman.

Second, the credibility of your record as evidence is enhanced by its being made at the time of the incident. Credibility is essential to the reliability of the record as evidence of what occurred. Using indelible ink or typeface reassures the court that the entry has not been subsequently altered in any way. You must, therefore, avoid using pencil or a computer entry system that does not use a time stamp or some other method to ensure that the entry cannot be altered without a trace. Altering a record is seen as a serious matter and can result in prosecution, dismissal and removal from the nursing register.

Scenario 9.7

Student who altered record is jailed

A student who faked her birth delivery figures at a Southampton hospital to boost her hopes of qualifying as a midwife was jailed for six months (Hampshire and Isle of Wight Counter Fraud Team, 2007). The student altered computer records at the hospital to show that she had gained sufficient experience to qualify in her profession. Using colleagues' passwords, she changed the details to convince her supervisor that she had overseen almost 30 births more than she actually had.

Records must be clear and unambiguous

Records are an essential tool in the continuity of care. Care to be implemented and progress made must be clearly stated. The record is also likely to be read by non-nursing and non-medical persons. Under the Data Protection Act 1998, patients have the right to access records and obtain an explanation of their contents. The Human Rights Act 1998 (schedule 1, part 1, article 8) gives a separate right of access both to patients and in some respects to relatives, where this affects their right to respect for a private and family life. In *Gaskin v UK* [1990], the European Court of Human Rights emphasised the need for specific justification for preventing individuals from having access to information that forms part of their private and family life.

Access to health records

A legal right of access to health records is given to living people, whether their records are computerised or manually created (handwritten), under the provisions of the Data Protection Act 1998 and its regulations. The right of access applies equally to all records regardless of when they were made. Limited statutory rights of access to the records of deceased patients still exist in the Access to Health Records Act 1990.

Access rights under the Data Protection Act 1998

Patients have a right to be informed as to whether personal data about them is being processed, including being obtained, recorded or held, and why (for more detail, see Chapter 10 on confidentiality). Patients have a right of access to health records that:

- are about them and from which they can be identified;
- consist of information relating to their physical or mental health or condition;
- have been made by or on behalf of a health professional in connection with their care.

Where access is agreed, the health record must be communicated to the patient in an intelligible form. That will often require the person responsible for the record meeting with the patient to explain the content and any technical or cryptic remarks or abbreviations that may be within it. Patients are entitled to a permanent copy of the information and this must also be accompanied by an explanation of any terms that are unintelligible to them. Where the person considers that the record or part of it is inaccurate, they can seek a correction.

You are not obliged to accept the patient's opinion or version of events, but you must ensure that the record indicates the patient's view and provide them with a copy of the correction or appended note. These arrangements must indicate why the alteration was made to avoid any allegation of tampering with the record.

If the person remains dissatisfied with their record, they may take the matter to court. The courts have the power to require that inaccurate data and any expression of opinion based on them are corrected or removed. The court may also require that the records be supplemented by a statement of the true facts, and that third parties be notified of any corrections.

Applications for access

Nothing in the Act prevents nurses from giving patients access to their records on an informal and voluntary basis, provided no other provisions of the Act preventing disclosure are breached. Indeed, the Data Protection Act 1998 calls for you to work in partnership with patients in an open and informal way, so that, if access to a record is requested, there are no surprises for patients. Formal applications for access must be in writing and accompanied by the appropriate fee.

Any patient is entitled to seek access to their health records. Where the patient is a child, any person with parental responsibility may apply independently. Where the child's parents live apart and have parental responsibility, they may individually apply to see their child's record. Where this occurs the other parent does not need to be told.

In *Gillick v West Norfolk and Wisbech AHA* [1986], the House of Lords held that, where a child is competent to make their own decisions about treatment, they are entitled to the same degree of confidentiality as an adult patient. Where access to a competent child's record is requested, it can only be granted if the child consents.

Competent children and young people may, of course, seek access to their own health records, and any patient may authorise a third party, such as a relative or legal representative, to seek access on their behalf.

Requests for access are made to the person in charge of keeping the records, known under the Data Protection Act 1998 as the data controller. The decision about disclosure is made by the appropriate health professional. This person would be the health professional currently or most recently respo~~~~~~ ~~ ~~~ ~~~~~~~~~ ~~ ~~~ patient. Access must be given promptly and, in any e~~~~ *DOCUMENTATION* f the fee and a clear request. Where access is given, t~~~~~~~~~~~~~~~~~~~~~~~~~~~ ess again until a reasonable time interval has elapsed. 1 *Q4 prof + legal* long this would be and it must be assessed on a case-l *issues associated* e patient has received no further treatment in the int *with record keeping* ss would seem unreasonable. *(disclosure)*

Information that cannot be disclosed

The right of access does not include information that would identify some other person mentioned in the record. This information cannot be released unless:

- the third party is a health professional who has compiled or contributed to the health records or who has been involved in the care of the patient;
- the other individual gives consent to the disclosure of that information; or
- it is reasonable to dispense with that third party's consent.

Where the record includes information from other identifiable sources, it is advisable to distinguish this information in the records when the information is entered, in order to avoid inadvertent disclosure. It is still necessary to disclose as much of the information in the records as is possible, but you must ensure that you:

- omit names and identifying particulars from the records before disclosure; and
- ensure that the information is genuinely anonymous.

You are not required to approach a third party for consent to disclosure, although you may wish to in some circumstances.

Harm

Access must not be given to any information that, in the opinion of the appropriate health professional, would be likely to cause serious harm to the patient or another person. The decision about likely harm must be taken by the appropriate health professional. This exemption does not justify withholding comments in the records because patients may find them upsetting.

Scenario 9.8

Refusal to grant access to a health record

In R (on the application of S) v Plymouth City Council [2002], a mother whose son was the subject of guardianship under the Mental Health Act was refused access to his health and social services record. She argued that she needed access to decide if she should accept or object to his continued guardianship order. The court granted access and it then emerged that the record contained uncomplimentary remarks about the woman.

Children

The Act does not allow disclosure of information prohibited in legislation concerning adoption records and reports, statements of a child's special educational needs and parental order records and reports. None of these exemptions apply where the disclosure is required by law, or where it is necessary for the purposes of establishing, exercising or defending legal rights.

Access to records of deceased patients

The Data Protection Act 1998 does not cover the records of deceased patients. Statutory rights of access are granted within the provisions of the Access to Health Records Act 1990.

Any person with a claim arising from the death of a patient has a right of access to information covered by the 1990 Act, where this information is directly relevant to that claim. The information that can be accessed is, however, restricted to that covered by the Access to Health Records Act 1990, that is, manually created (handwritten) health records made since 1 November 1991.

Use of jargon and abbreviations

The temptation to use jargon and abbreviations as a form of professional shorthand is compelling for busy overworked health staff. However, the risk of miscommunication increases dramatically by using this shorthand.

Activity 9.3

Abbreviations and jargon

In a group, write down individual lists of abbreviations and technical jargon you have used or read during your clinical placements. Now pass the lists among the other group members and ask them to explain what they understand by the terms and abbreviations. Did you all come to the same definitions and meaning of the terms?

An outline answer is given at the end of the chapter.

A combination of shorthand instructions and poor handwriting led to the death of a patient. The patient was taking 2mg of warfarin daily. When reviewed, the GP wrote 'same' on the card. The receptionist mistook the 's' as a 5 and the rest of the word as mg, resulting in the patient being given 5mg of warfarin daily. He died from a massive haemorrhage some three weeks later (Marsh and Narain, 2003).

Although under considerable work pressure, nurses must not use abbreviations or jargon. The risks are too great and misinterpretation by staff and patients is common.

Scenario 9.9

Misinterpretation of abbreviations

Wright (2003) reported an incident where a member of nursing staff who, when he saw DOA on a patient's notes, told the enquiring relative that the patient was 'dead on arrival' at hospital. This was the meaning of the acronym in A & E, where he usually worked. On the ward, however, DOA meant 'date of admission' and the patient was very much alive.

Jargon is also used to convey offensive remarks unrelated to patient care. Brindley (2003) reported that a GP wrote 'She's mad', along with a cartoon drawing, on a set of notes. Other cryptic acronyms are more offensive. Examples include CLL or 'chronic low life', FLK for 'funny-looking kid', often explained by JLD or 'just like dad'. The temptation to use such acronyms is always there.

Remember, in litigation your records will be subject to rigorous scrutiny. There is no right to withhold any part of the record from the court. Having to explain under cross-examination that the entry GPO meant you thought the patient was 'good for parts only' will be at best embarrassing and at worst fatal to your case. Evidentially, the first impression the court has of you is from your notes. Cryptic comments have no place in records. If records are not professional, the assumption is that neither is your care and your credibility as a witness is greatly diminished.

Records must be accurate

To confirm the chronology of record entries, each entry must be identified with date (day, month and year) and time (using the 24-hour clock) and signed with the professional's name printed legibly underneath the signature together with their position. Initials for entries must not be used, as it is vital to be able to identify the member of staff if a complaint is made.

Scenario 9.10

Ten minutes of unexplained delay

In *Richards v Swansea NHS Trust* [2007], a child suffered from cerebral palsy and argued that it was as the result of delaying, at the time of his birth, the emergency caesarean that had occurred some 50 minutes after it was considered necessary. Professional guidance states that it must occur within 30 minutes and the judge was content to grant the trust a period of 40 minutes, but the trust and care team had to justify the extra 10-minute delay. As they were unable to demonstrate what call on their time there was during that 10-minute period, the judge said he had no alternative but to find for the patient.

Errors

All alterations must be made by scoring out with a single line that does not completely obscure the error. Correcting fluid must not be used. This removes any suggestion of wrongdoing or attempting to cover up an incident. The struck-out error should be followed by the dated, timed and signed correct entry. No blank lines or spaces that could facilitate entries being added at a later date should be left between entries.

Pressure of work

It may be argued that pressure of work was such that it reduced the nurse's ability to maintain the usual standard of care. Such situations have been called 'battlefield situations', in which resources are so stretched that a court has to accept that the expected level of the standard of care has to be reduced (*Wilsher v Essex HA* [1988]). In these situations, the court can order the disclosure of other patients' records to see how busy the ward was at the time.

Pressure of work

In *Deacon v McVicar* (1984), a woman argued that she had received negligent care causing her harm. The hospital argued that the evening of the incident was a singularly busy one, with several emergency cases draining available resources. The court ordered that the records of all other patients on the ward that evening be released to the court to see how busy the unit was. They showed that it was an exceptionally busy evening with many emergencies overstretching the staff and resources available.

Contemporaneous record entries

Record entries need to be written at the time of, or as soon as possible after, the events to which they relate. Contemporaneous recording is vital as it adds to the reliability of the entry and means that, with the leave of the court, you can refer to the record when giving evidence. Contemporaneous altering of a record contributed to a finding of negligence in *Kent v Griffiths and Others* [2000]. Here, an emergency ambulance took some 30 minutes to arrive at an address, but the crew recorded the duration of the journey as 9 minutes. The judge held that the record had been contemporaneously falsified and found for the patient.

The record should demonstrate the chronology of events and of all significant consultations, assessments, observations, decisions, interventions and outcomes. Reports and results should be seen, evaluated and signed by the practitioner before being filed in the patient records. This is the key to a good record. This is what a lawyer is going to try and pull apart in order to win a case. If the patient's condition remains the same, say so. In one case, a record entry stated, *6.30 a.m. sleeping peacefully, 8.40 a.m. dead* (Wright, 2003). In the cold light of a courtroom such an entry makes it look like the patient was not being properly monitored.

Records are never neutral

To be of use in evidence your records need to be thorough, otherwise they will act to your detriment. Records are never neutral; they will either support or condemn you.

The incomplete record

In *S (A Child) v Newcastle and North Tyneside HA* [2001], the negligent management of the latter stages of labour resulted in severe cerebral palsy. The judge's annoyance at the standard of record keeping is clear from his comments:

> It is important to emphasise at this early stage that unhappily the evidence was, in certain important respects, incomplete. The clinical records of this labour are not full and no records at all appear between 4 a.m. and 10.15 a.m. Each of these might be regarded as critical periods. Unhappily who ever did take over from [the midwife] singularly failed to complete the partogram, that is the record of the labour, which is effectively devoid of useful information.

The importance of personal details

The patient's personal details are every bit as important as the care plan and progress entries. The Audit Commission (2002) found that the average NHS Trust wastes some £20,000 per year on redirected mail due to incorrectly addressed home or GP details that have been recorded in the notes or on the computer system. Missing details also reduce the quality of patient care by disrupting communication between the patients, their families and health staff, causing missed outpatient appointments and losing potentially critical information about the patient. It is important to check details with patients to ensure that personal information is up to date.

Records need to be communicated

Your records are a crucial means of communicating with colleagues. It is essential for effective patient care that records are used and communicated. Where tragedy occurs in health settings, the resulting inquiry report repeatedly cites a failure of communication as a cause. It is a recurring theme in mental health inquiries (Anderson, 2003) and in child death inquiries (DH, 2003a). Records are not a paper exercise. Nurses must communicate the contents and findings of their records to other members of the care team to ensure that concerns and risks are monitored and minimised.

Scenario 9.13

The consequences of a failure to communicate a record entry

In *Gauntlett v Northampton HA* [1985], a patient gave her visiting husband a box of matches saying 'Take these because I'll set fire to myself'. Her husband handed the matches to the charge nurse, who failed to record or communicate the concern. Four days later the patient set fire to the tee shirt she was wearing, burning herself badly.

Keeping records secure

All NHS records are public records _____ _____ of the Public Records Act 1958 (sections 3(1)–(2)). The _____ ___ _nd all NHS organisations have a duty under this Act to _____ ___ _____ _ith_re keeping and eventual disposal of all records. Chief _ _____ _____ managers of all NHS organisations are personally accountabl_ _____ _eeping of records.

Activity 9.4

Security of patient records

What measures must you take to ensure the safety and security of patient records?

Now read below for further information.

Under the Public Records Act, nurses are accountable for any records that they create or use in the course of their duties. You have a duty to ensure that records are kept safe and secure by:

- ensuring the physical security of such records, keeping them locked away when not required;

- ensuring that records and their binders are in a good state so that information is held securely, loose-leaf information ~~such as test results~~ ecured, and information cannot be lost or mislaid
- maintaining security of access to info~~rmation~~ ~~ds by~~ ~~s~~uring that they cannot be inadvertently read by ~~others~~
- maintaining a written log of incoming ~~and~~ ~~records through the~~ se of a tracing system that allows for the ph~~ysical~~ ~~location~~

[handwritten margin note: DOCUMENTATION & professional + legal issues associated with records]

Putting the record straight

The Audit Commission (2002) found that subjecting records to a regular audit is the best way to ensure high-quality record keeping.

Activity 9.5

Audit of records

Having read this chapter, if you were to audit your record entries, what key standards would you wish to meet?

Now read below for further information.

In their advice sheet on record keeping, the NMC (2007) recommends the following content for nursing records. The information in patient records must:

- be factual, consistent and accurate;
- be written in such a way that the meaning is clear;
- be recorded as soon as possible after an event has occurred;
- be recorded clearly and indelibly;
- be recorded so that any justifiable alterations or additions are dated, timed and signed in such a way that the original entry can still be read clearly;
- be accurately dated, timed and signed, with the signature printed alongside the first entry, where this is a written record, and attributed to a named person in an identifiable role for electronic records;
- not include abbreviations, jargon, meaningless phrases, irrelevant speculation or offensive or subjective statements;
- be readable when photocopied or scanned;
- be recorded, wherever possible, with the involvement of the patient;
- be recorded in terms that the patient can understand;
- be in chronological order;
- identify risks or problems that have arisen and the action taken to rectify them;
- give a full account of the assessment and the care that has been planned and provided;
- provide relevant information about the condition of the patient;
- provide evidence that you have discharged your duty of care;
- provide a record of any arrangements that have been made for the continuing care of a patient.

You are also required to make more frequent entries for patients who:

- have complex problems;
- are vulnerable or at risk of harm or abuse;
- require more intensive care than normal;
- are confused and disoriented or generally give cause for concern.

| C H A P T E R | S U M M A R Y |

- Record keeping is a basic nursing duty.
- Records provide evidence of involvement with patients.
- Record provide a plan of care for a patient and are crucial in monitoring progress and communicating concerns.
- Records also have a vital role in protecting nurses from litigation.
- If it is not written down it is difficult to prove it happened.
- Records must be thorough, contemporaneous and clear.
- Expressions of dissent must be recorded.
- Records must corroborate discussions with colleagues.
- Records must be communicated to be effective.
- Records subject to audit have a higher standard of record keeping.
- Good record keeping will demonstrate that you have met your legal and professional obligations and discharged your duty of care.

Activities: brief outline answer

9.3 Abbreviations and jargon (page 169)

The temptation to use jargon and abbreviations as a form of professional shorthand is compelling for busy, overworked health staff. However, as this activity demonstrates, the risk of miscommunication increases dramatically by using this shorthand.

Here are some other examples:

- UBI: unexplained beer injury;
- NQR: not quite right;
- GOK: God only knows.

Knowledge review

Now that you've worked through the chapter, how would you rate your knowledge of the following topics?

	Good	Adequate	Poor
1. Defining a health record.			
2. The purposes of nurses keeping patient records.			
3. The style and content of a nursing record.			
4. The elements of good record keeping.			
5. The role of audit in raising the standard of record keeping.			

	Good	Adequate	Poor
6. The right of access to records of patients who are living compared with access to the records of patients who have died.			

Where you are not confident in your knowledge of a topic, what will you do next?

Further reading

Department of Health (DH) (2006) *Records Management: NHS code of practice.* London: The Stationery Office.

Nursing and Midwifery Council (NMC) (2007) *NMC Record Keeping Guidance.* London: NMC.

Useful websites

www.dh.gov.uk Department of Health.

www.nmc-uk.org Nursing and Midwifery Council.

Chapter 10

Confidentiality

Chapter aims

By the end of this chapter you will be able to:

* discuss the rationale for imposing a duty of confidence on registered nurses and midwives;
* outline three spheres of the duty of confidence that registered nurses and midwives are subject to;
* compare the scope of the legal, professional and contractual obligation of confidence;
* describe the circumstances that would allow you to disclose confidential patient information;
* explain three ways in which the duty of confidence may be modified by statute;
* discuss the measures nurses must take to ensure that confidential patient information is disclosed with appropriate care.

Introduction

Maintaining the confidentiality of a patient's health information is a fundamental element of professional conduct and ethical practice for all registered nurses. The relationship between nurse and patient is essential for proper assessment and care that is largely based on a patient's personal history of their health problem. Patients pass on sensitive information relating to their health and other matters as part of their desire to receive treatment. They do so in confidence and expect you to respect their privacy by ensuring the confidentiality of the information they give.

To ensure the highest standard of conduct and ethical practice in relation to the protection of health information, a duty of confidence is imposed on all staff, volunteers and contractors within the NHS.

Activity 10.1

Defining confidentiality

Before you begin reading about the nurse's duty of confidence to the patient, write down what you consider the term confidentiality means.

An outline answer is given at the end of the chapter.

Duty of confidence

A duty of confidence arises when one person discloses information to another in circumstances where it is reasonable to expect that the information will be held in confidence.

For nurses, there are three key spheres to the duty that come together to reassure patients that the confidentiality of their health information will be respected (see Figure 10.1).

1. A duty to respect patient confidentiality that is a specific requirement linked to disciplinary procedures in all NHS employment contracts and underpinned by the NHS code of practice on confidentiality (DH, 2003c).
2. A legal duty that is derived from case law and supplemented by statute law (*Cornelius v De Taranto* [2001]).
3. A professional duty established by *The Code: Standards of Conduct, Performance and ethics for nurses* and *midwives* (NMC, 2008).

Figure 10.1: The three spheres of the duty of confidence owed by registered nurses and midwives.

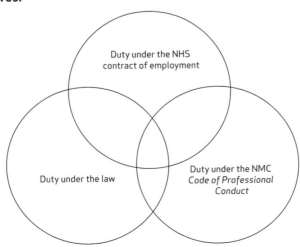

However, the duty of confidence is not absolute. There will be occasions when confidential information about a patient will need to be disclosed to others. Such a disclosure must be to an appropriate person and comply with the requirements of your contractual, professional and legal duty of confidence, or you will be called to account and face sanctions for breaching confidentiality.

It is essential, therefore, that you:

- understand the scope of the duty of confidence owed to the patients in your care; and
- only disclose information given in confidence where it is right and proper to do so.

Activity 10.2

The need for a duty of confidence

You have seen that a duty of confidence is imposed on nurses requiring them to respect the confidentiality of patient information. Write down why you think it is necessary for nurses to be subject to a legal, professional and contractual duty of confidence to their patients.

An outline answer is given at the end of the chapter.

The scope of the duty

The contractual duty of confidence

In recognition of the need to protect patient information and maintain the confidentiality of health information, all contracts of employment in the NHS must contain a clause that imposes a duty of confidence on all staff and stresses that disciplinary action will result if that duty is breached (DH, 2003c). Similarly, all contracts with outside agencies and arrangements with volunteers and others – including student nurses – who undertake work or placements with the NHS must also include a clause imposing a duty of confidence.

In order to discharge this duty, all staff and students will need to show that they have fulfilled their responsibilities by ensuring that:

- they do not disclose confidential patient information through inappropriate means, such as gossiping;
- when they seek advice about a patient's care and treatment with a colleague, they do so in private so that confidentiality is not inadvertently breached;
- they accurately record information received from and about their patients;
- they keep patient information and records private and physically secure;
- they only access information for the patients in their care;
- they only disclose patient information to an appropriate source in accordance with the NHS code of practice on confidentiality, the requirements of the law and the NMC *Code*.

Scenario 10.1

Celebrity records

When a former England and Newcastle United manager was admitted to Newcastle General Hospital to have surgery, his records were accessed by staff who were not involved in his clinical care but who were curious to find out about their footballing hero (*Northern Echo*, 2006).

Scenario 10.1 continued

Officials at the Trust became suspicious when security reports showed that there had been inappropriate access to the Trust's patient records system.

Staff are not permitted to look up patient records unless there is a direct medical need and disciplinary action was taken against ten members of staff at the hospital.

The duty extends to all patients, both past and present. Although there is no specific legal or professional requirement that states that a duty of confidence extends to deceased patients, the contractual duty imposed by the NHS extends confidentiality beyond the grave and includes those who have died.

The professional duty of confidence

The professional requirement for confidentiality is stipulated in the NMC's *Code* (2008) which states that a registered nurse must respect people's right to confidentiality.

Activity 10.3

The professional duty of confidence

Download and read the Nursing and Midwifery Council's explanatory note on Confidentiality (at www.nmc-uk.org), then

- outline the extent of a nurse's professional duty of confidence to patients;
- list the exceptions to that duty that would allow you to disclose information about a patient.

An outline answer is given at the end of the chapter.

This clause imposes on nurses a duty not to voluntarily disclose information gained in a professional capacity to a third party, and this is enforced by the threat of professional discipline. An explanatory paper by the NMC on professional conduct highlights a breach of confidentiality as a form of misconduct likely to result in removal from the register (NMC, 2004b).

Scenario 10.2

Inappropriate disclosure of patient information in breach of a nurse's professional duty of confidence

A specialist community public health nurse who had an affair with an ex-patient told him of an abortion his partner had undergone 19 years earlier (*Evening Gazette*, 2006). When asked where she had got the information from, she revealed that it had come from the woman's health record. The nurse admitted breaching confidentiality and was found guilty by a Conduct and Competence Committee of the NMC, who removed her name from the professional register.

Confidence and the law

As well as the professional duty of confidence there is a legal obligation on nurses to respect patients' confidences. The law relating to confidence is dealt with largely at common law. The obligation arises out of a general duty on everyone to keep confidential information secret (*Prince Albert v Strange* (1849)). That is, there is a public interest in keeping confidential information secret.

In order to establish a breach of confidence, three elements must be satisfied, as stated by Lord Keith in *Attorney General v Guardian Newspapers Ltd* [1987]:

1.   The information must have the necessary quality of confidence. That is, the information is not generally available or known. Information of a personal or intimate nature qualifies (*Stephens v Avery* [1988]) and this is very much the type of information nurses receive from their patients.
2.   The information has been imparted in circumstances giving rise to an obligation of confidence. The law has long recognised that particular relationships gave rise to a duty of confidence. These include priest and penitent, solicitor and client, and the nurse–patient relationship. The courts, however, have gone further and have extended the obligation to include situations where an obviously confidential document is wafted by an electric fan out of a window into a crowded street, or a private diary is dropped in a public place [or these days an email goes astray].
3.   The information has been divulged to a third person without the permission and to the detriment of the person originally communicating the information. An invasion of personal privacy will suffice (*Margaret, Duchess of Argyll v Duke of Argyll* [1967]). As it is in the public interest that medical confidences are kept secret, the court will regard an unwarranted disclosure of patient information as detrimental.

It can be seen that the very private nature of the information nurses are given by their patients and the trust generated by the nature of the nurse–patient relationship give rise to an obligation of confidence that the law seeks to protect. Consequently, the court will consider that an inappropriate disclosure of this information is bound to be detrimental to the patient and find that a breach of confidence has occurred.

Scenario 10.3

Breaching the common law duty of confidence to a patient

In *X v Y and Others* [1988], a health authority employee passed on to a newspaper information obtained from medical records of two patients who were HIV positive. The patients worked as doctors in the area and the newspaper wished to publish the details. The court granted the doctors an injunction preventing publication, holding that the public interest in preserving the confidentiality of hospital records outweighed any public interest in the freedom of the press, because victims of the disease ought not to be deterred by fear of discovery from going to hospital for treatment.

As well as a general duty of confidence established under the common law, there are a range of statutory provisions that limit or prohibit the use and disclosure of information in specific circumstances.

Data Protection Act 1998

The Data Protection Act 1998 implements a European Union directive on the protection of individuals with regard to the processing of personal data and on the free movement of such data (Directive 95/46/EC). The 1998 Act provides a framework that governs the so-called processing of personal data.

Personal data is defined under the Data Protection Act 1998 as data that relates to a living individual who can be identified:

- from that data; or
- from data and other information that may be in your possession.

This includes any expression of opinion about the individual and any indications of your intentions to the individual.

'Processing' is an umbrella term and includes:

- holding information about patients;
- obtaining information from patients or others about a patient;
- recording patient information;
- using the information;
- disclosing patient information.

The 1998 Act applies to all forms of media, including paper records, electronic records and images.

All processing of patient information must be fair and lawful and this will usually be the case where:

- the common law of confidentiality and any other applicable statutory restrictions on the use of information are complied with;
- the patient, known as the data subject, was not misled or deceived into giving the information;
- the patient is given basic information about who will process the data and for what purpose;
- in the case of personal health information, the conditions of schedules 2 and 3 of the Data Protection Act 1998 concerning sensitive data are met by ensuring that the information is necessary for medical purposes.

Human Rights Act 1998

Article 8 of the European Convention on Fundamental Rights and Freedoms establishes a right to respect for private and family life. This right emphasises the duty to protect the privacy of individuals and preserve the confidentiality of their health records. Article 8 is broad in scope and covers the collection, use and exchange of personal data as well as issues such as telephone tapping, parental access and the custody of children, the right to be free from noise and environmental pollution, and a person's right to express their identity and sexuality. Public authorities must preserve the individual's confidence when collecting and using personal data.

In *R (Robertson) v City of Wakefield Metropolitan Council* [2002], a man complained that his right to respect for a private life under article 8 of the European Convention on Human Rights was being infringed by his local council as they were selling to commercial companies personal details that he was required to provide for inclusion on the electoral roll. These companies were using the information for direct marketing.

The Court held that article 8 was breached by the council. In determining whether article 8 was engaged it was necessary to take into account not just the information that was disclosed, but also the use to which it would be put. Where names and addresses were to be passed on to commercial companies for direct marketing purposes, this amounted to an interference with the right to private life.

Exceptions to the obligation of confidence

Neither the professional nor legal duties of confidentiality are absolute and they are subject to a range of exceptions that justify disclosure. It is important that nurses are aware of these exceptions in order to avoid a charge of professional misconduct and liability for breach of confidence.

The NMC, in clause 5 of the *Code* (2008), leaves the decision to divulge a confidence with the registered nurse by viewing it as a matter of professional judgement. Yet little specific guidance is given on circumstances in which disclosure is justified. No guidance is given on the difference between a power to disclose, where a nurse can consider all the circumstances and decide if it is appropriate to divulge information, and a duty to disclose, where, regardless of circumstances, the law requires disclosure.

Activity 10.4

Disclosing information about patients

The duty of confidence owed by a nurse is not absolute. There will be times when it will be appropriate to disclose information about a patient.

Consider circumstances where you would think it was appropriate to divulge information about patients in your care.

An outline answer is given at the end of the chapter.

Consent of the patient

Permission to disclose confidential information from the person who originally imparted it is the starting presumption in law and an obvious exception. The courts generally require this consent to disclosure be in the form of an explicit consent, preferably signed by the patient (*Cornelius v De Taranto* [2001]). This ruling also reflects the requirements of the Data Protection Act 1998. The consent exception is only valid if the person knows exactly what information is to be disclosed and who is to receive the information.

The requirements for obtaining explicit consent from patients for the disclosure of personal health information are:

- be honest and clear about the information to be disclosed and the reason for disclosure, allowing patients to seek as much detail as they require to make a free choice;
- give patients an opportunity to talk to someone they trust and ask questions;
- allow the patient reasonable time to reach a decision;
- be prepared to explain any form that the patient may be required to sign;
- explain that consent can be refused or withdrawn at any time;
- ensure that you note that consent has been received in a patient's health record or by using a consent form signed by the patient.

Disclosure for care and treatment purposes

An area where a nurse might exercise professional judgement and disclose confidential information is with those directly involved in the care of the patient.

Confidentiality is allowed to be breached where information is shared with other nurses concerned with the clinical care of the patient. This exception also covers doctors and others for whom the information provided is necessary for the performance of their duties. These professionals are also bound by a duty of confidentiality. To require an express consent from a patient each time a patient's case was discussed would be impractical and even detrimental to the patient.

Where patients have consented to healthcare, research has consistently shown that they are content for information to be disclosed in order to provide that healthcare (NHS Information Authority, 2002).

It is still essential that you ensure that patients understand how their information is to be used to support their healthcare and that they have no objections. To ensure this, you must:

- check where practicable that information leaflets on patient confidentiality and information disclosure have been read and understood by the patient;
- make it clear to patients why personal health information is recorded and why health records need to be accessed by other health professionals;
- make it clear to patients why you need to share their health information with others;
- ensure that patients have no concerns about how you will use their personal information;
- answer any questions the patient may have or direct the patient to someone who can answer their questions;
- respect the rights of patients to request access to their health records.

Where the patient has no objections, consent can be implied, provided that the information is shared no more widely than with those directly concerned with the care and treatment of the individual. Wide disclosure to any doctor or nurse is not justified.

Scenario 10.4

The limit to the clinical family

In *Cornelius v De Taranto* [2001], a teacher who claimed to be suffering from work-related stress saw a psychiatrist privately as part of gathering evidence against her employer. The psychiatrist sent a copy of her medico-legal report to the teacher's GP and a general consultant psychiatrist, as well as to her solicitor. Mrs Cornelius sued for breach of confidence. The Court of Appeal held that there was a breach of confidence and that Mrs Cornelius had not expressly consented to the dissemination of the report. The report had nothing to do with her treatment, so dissemination to other health professionals could not be justified on therapeutic grounds. The doctor could not rely on an implied consent in these circumstances.

Patients who refuse consent to disclose treatment information

Patients have the right to be informed that they can object to the disclosure of confidential information that identifies them.

Where a patient refuses to allow information to be disclosed to other health professionals involved in providing care, it could mean that the care that can be provided is limited and in some circumstances it might not be possible to offer treatment.

Patients must be told if their decisions to refuse to allow disclosure of treatment information will have implications for the provision of care or treatment. Health professionals cannot treat patients safely or provide continuity of care without having relevant information about a patient's condition and medical history.

Disclosing information when a patient specifically asks you to do so

When a health professional is asked by a patient to pass on confidential information about them, the court regards this as a binding obligation. In *C v C* [1946], Justice Lewis considered the refusal of a sexually transmitted disease clinic to divulge information about a patient despite his request for disclosure. The judge held that, while it was important that proper secrecy be observed in sexually transmitted disease clinics, those considerations did not justify a health professional refusing to divulge confidential information to a named person when asked by the patient to do so. In the circumstances of this case the information should have been given, and in all cases where the circumstances are similar there is no breach of confidence in giving the information asked for.

Activity 10.5

Share with Care

Download a copy of *Share with Care: People's views on consent and confidentiality of patient information* (NHS Information Authority, 2002) by following the link on the book's website. Read and consider what the report discovered about patients' views on health professionals disclosing their personal information.

An outline answer is given at the end of the chapter.

Disclosing information without specific consent

The Department of Health advises that there are a number of exceptions allowing disclosure to appropriate sources without the consent of the patient (DH, 2003c). These exceptions act as a useful aid to nurses when making a judgement about disclosing information concerning a patient.

Where a patient is incapable of receiving information or of consenting to disclosure, disclosure of care and treatment information to the client's relative or main carer may be judged to be appropriate. Similarly, disclosure to appropriate sources would be allowed in cases of the suspected abuse of dependent elderly people and children under vulnerable adult and child protection procedures (DH, 1999b, 2002).

Disclosure in the public interest

A major defence used by individuals who have had to justify the disclosure of confidential information has been that disclosure was necessary in the public interest. The courts accept that, when a case concerning the disclosure of confidential information comes before them, they are required to strike a balance between two competing interests:

- the public interest in keeping confidential information secret; and
- the public interest in allowing disclosure.

The public interest exception covers a broad range of situations that allow for confidential information to be disclosed without the consent of the patient. These situations include:

- disclosure in the interests of justice;
- disclosure for the public good;
- disclosure to protect a third party;
- disclosure to prevent or detect a serious crime.

Disclosure in the interests of justice

Unlike lawyers, nurses do not have a privileged relationship with their patients. A court has the power to order disclosure of confidential matters if it is in the interest of justice, and refusing to do so would result in conviction for contempt of court. For example, in *Attorney General v Mulholland* [1963], two journalists refused before a tribunal to name or describe the sources of information in articles written by them, which the chairman of the tribunal certified were relevant to the inquiry. One of the journalists was sentenced to six and the other to three months' imprisonment for contempt. On appeal, the court confirmed that the questions were relevant and necessary to the tribunal's inquiry; thus there was no privilege and the sentences would stand.

In exercising this power the court must be satisfied that disclosure will satisfy the interests of justice. Where this is not the case they can refuse to order disclosure. For example, in *D v National Society for the Prevention of Cruelty to Children* [1977], the NSPCC received a complaint from an informant about the alleged maltreatment of a girl aged 14 months. That evening an inspector from the society called at the parents' home and enquired about the baby. The mother, who was very upset, called the family doctor, who found the baby to be healthy and unharmed. The family demanded to be told the name of the informant. When the inspector refused to give it, the family brought legal proceedings to reveal the identity of the informant. The House of Lords held that the importance of preserving confidentiality for the protection of children overrode the requirement that the mother should be given the information she sought in order to pursue her claim.

Nurses, therefore, could be required by the courts to disclose information about their patients both in the form of written statements and as oral evidence, where this is necessary in the interests of justice.

Disclosure for the public good

There may be circumstances where the public interest is served by disclosing information even though no crime has been committed or court action taken. This might include disclosing information to a regulatory body such as the NMC. For example, in *Woolgar v Chief Constable of Sussex* [2000], a nurse was interviewed under caution by the police following a patient's death over alleged drug misuse. The information obtained was insufficient to bring charges. The police passed the tapes to the nursing regulatory body, which was investigating the nurse, and she claimed a breach of confidence. The Court of Appeal held that comments made in police interviews were confidential and remained so even if not used in criminal proceedings. However, disclosure to a regulatory body could be justified in the absence of consent if it was necessary for the public good to allow the regulatory body to properly investigate the allegations against the nurse.

Disclosure to protect a third party

The law accepts that there may be circumstances where disclosure of confidential information is necessary in order to protect a third party, particularly where this concerns a vulnerable adult or child. The nurse would need to consider all the circumstances and use their professional judgement, informed by reference to the common law, to decide if the public interest in protecting the third party outweighed the public interest in keeping confidential information secret.

For example, in *Re L (Care Proceedings: Disclosure to Third Party)* [2000], a paediatric nurse sought an injunction preventing a local authority passing information about her mental health problem to the nursing regulatory body following care proceedings concerning her and her child. The court allowed the disclosure, holding that the right of the nurse and her child to confidentiality had to be balanced against the public interests in protecting others from a nurse whose fitness to practise had been called into doubt.

Disclosure to prevent or detect a serious crime

There may be circumstances where a nurse is made aware that a patient has committed or intends to commit a crime. Before disclosing such information, it will be necessary for the health professional to weigh the seriousness of the crime against the countervailing public interest in maintaining patient confidentiality.

For example, in *W v Egdell* [1990], Dr Egdell had been commissioned by W's solicitor to prepare a report for his upcoming appeal against detention under the Mental Health Act 1983. W had been an in-patient at a special hospital for ten years after he shot five people and was now seeking discharge or relocation to a less secure unit. His consultant psychiatrist supported W's appeal as he felt he had made good progress. However, Dr Egdell's report strongly opposed his relocation and pointed out W's continued interest in firearms and explosives. On receiving the report, W's solicitor withdrew the appeal, which prompted Dr Egdell to send a copy to the medical director of the hospital as he felt the patient was deceiving his doctors. W then sued for breach of confidence.

The court held that Dr Egdell's duty of confidence to W had to be weighed against the public interests in preventing crime. Dr Egdell was justified in taking this course of action as W posed a real risk to public safety, and the medical team at the hospital were entitled to full information relating to his dangerousness.

It can be seen from *Egdell* that disclosure is justified where the crime represents a real risk to public safety. That is, there must be a need to prevent or detect a serious crime to justify breaching patient confidentiality, as the countervailing public interest in maintaining sensitive health information would generally outweigh disclosure.

It is very interesting to contrast the disclosure in *W v Egdell* [1990] with the earlier case of *X v Y and Others* [1988], where two doctors in general practice had their HIV status revealed to a national newspaper by employees of a health authority. Here, the court held that there was a breach of confidentiality, as there was no public interest to justify overriding the duty of confidence owed to the doctors.

Where a nurse believes they are justified in disclosing information about a patient, that disclosure must be to an appropriate source. Indeed, Lord Justice Bingham, in *W v Egdell* [1990], stressed that, while the doctor was right to pass on information to other doctors in Broadmoor about W's dangerousness, he could not lawfully sell the contents of his report to a newspaper. Nor could he, without a breach of the law as well as professional etiquette, discuss the case in a learned article or in his memoirs or in gossiping with friends, unless he took steps to conceal the identity of the patient.

Is there a duty to warn of risk of physical harm?

In one American case, the concept of disclosure in the public interest was taken a stage further when a counsellor was successfully sued for failing to disclose information about a serious risk of physical harm to a client's ex-girlfriend on the grounds of client confidentiality. In *Tarasoff v Regents of the University of California* (1976), Tatiana

Tarasoff was killed by her ex-boyfriend and the University of California was sued by her parents. The California Supreme Court heard the case twice and extended the duty to warn on each occasion.

In the first trial they held that privilege ends where public peril begins. In the second, that a therapist has a duty to use reasonable care to protect potential victims. The *Tarasoff* case created a new cause of action in negligence in the United States.

Such has been the impact of the case in America that so-called *Tarasoff* warnings are routinely issued by psychiatrists and psychologists, warning potential victims of the threat towards them.

There is yet to be a similar case before the British courts. Little authoritative guidance is available on whether *Tarasoff* warnings are required to avoid liability in negligence by nurses and others in the UK. Any trial on the issue would largely depend on the legal proximity of the potential victim to the nurse. If the person is another patient of the nurse's, then a duty to warn is probably owed. If the person is a close relative of the patient and the nurse adopts a holistic or family-centred approach to care, it is argued that a duty would also exist. However, if the potential victim is an unidentified member of the public or someone the nurse does not know, no duty to warn will arise.

This was certainly held to be the case in *Palmer v Tees HA* (2000). Here, it was claimed that the health authority had been negligent in failing to diagnose the real and substantial risk that an outpatient in their care would sexually abuse children. The patient abducted and murdered a child and her mother sued the health authority for failing to warn the public of the risk he posed. However, the judge held that, where it was alleged that a defendant was responsible for the action of a third party, then that required a special class of person at risk, not an unidentified category.

Therefore, as the identity of the victim was not known to the health authority, it did not owe a duty of care. In seeking to expand on his judgment, the judge added that a health authority had no general immunity from an action of this sort if the case demanded it. If there had been any identifiable special factors that could have put the victim above other members of the public, the outcome may well have been different. Hence, if a person known to a health professional is identified as being at risk of harm from the criminal act of another patient, there probably exists a duty to warn.

Activity 10.6

Breach of confidentiality

You are working in a busy A & E department when, at about 2 a.m., a man presents himself with a wound to his left leg. He has apparently driven to the hospital on his own. He will not give any information about how he sustained this injury and he smells strongly of alcohol. He wants to be treated as soon as possible and then go home. Following an examination by the casualty officer, it becomes apparent that he has sustained a gunshot wound.

On your way to the reception area, you are approached by a police officer. He asks you if you have had a patient admitted with injuries to his leg. No one else is available to speak to the officer as they are all busy with a victim of a serious road traffic collision.

Discuss whether you would be justified in disclosing the name of the patient to the police officer.

An outline answer is given at the end of the chapter.

Statutes that modify the duty of confidence

There are three ways in which a statute can modify the duty of confidence owed by a nurse. The statute might:

1. reinforce the common law duty of confidence by providing penalties for unjustified disclosure;
2. empower the health professional to disclose information in specific circumstances if they consider it appropriate to do so; or
3. require the health professional to disclose information under specific circumstances, leaving you with no choice but to pass on the information.

Statutes that reinforce the common law duty of confidence

Information about sexually transmitted infections is considered particularly sensitive and private, and you should never assume that patients are happy for this information to be shared unless it has a direct and significant bearing on their healthcare. To ensure that confidential information regarding sexually transmitted infections remains private, the general duty of confidence is reinforced by the provisions of the AIDS (Control) Act 1987, the National Health Service (Venereal Diseases) Regulations 1974, the National Health Service Act 1977 and the National Health Service Trusts and Primary Care Trusts (Sexually Transmitted Diseases) Directions 2000. Under these provisions, every NHS Trust and Primary Care Trust must take all necessary steps to ensure that any information capable of identifying an individual examined or treated for any sexually transmitted infection, including HIV and AIDS, shall not be disclosed except:

- where there is explicit consent to do so;
- for the purpose of communicating that information to a medical practitioner, or to a person employed under the direction of a medical practitioner in connection with the treatment of persons suffering from such disease or the prevention of the spread thereof; and
- for the purpose of such treatment or prevention.

Similarly, the provisions of the Human Fertilisation and Embryology Act 1990 and the Human Fertilisation and Embryology (Disclosure of Information) Act 1992 apply restrictions on disclosure concerning fertilisation and embryo treatment where individuals can be identified. The explicit consent of the person is usually required before disclosure can be authorised unless it concerns:

- the provision of treatment services, or any other description of medical, surgical or obstetric services, for the individual giving the consent;
- the carrying out of an audit of clinical practice; or
- the auditing of accounts.

Statutes that empower the health professional to disclose information

The provisions of such statutes give the health professional the power to disclose. It is for the health professional to decide whether in all the circumstances it is appropriate to disclose the information.

Under the Health and Social Care Act 2001, section 60 allows the Secretary of State to specify circumstances in which it would be lawful for confidential information to be disclosed where the common law exemptions allowing disclosure are not clear. For example, the first regulations made under this provision allow for the use of information to create and monitor cancer registers, and for the surveillance and monitoring of communicable diseases that represent a risk to public health (The Health Service (Control of Patient Information) Regulations (SI 2002/1438) 2002).

Section 60 of the Health and Social Care Act 2001 also provides a power to ensure that patient identifiable information that is required to support a range of work, such as clinical audit, record validation and research, can be used without the consent of patients.

Other examples include:

- the Crime and Disorder Act 1998, section 115, which allows for disclosure of information to the police, local authorities or health authorities where the disclosure is necessary or expedient for the purposes of that Act, such as, for example, the prevention of crime or disorder;
- the Anti-Terrorism, Crime and Security Act 2001, section 17, which allows disclosure to be made for fairly broad purposes relating to criminal investigation and prosecution.

Statutes that require the health professional to disclose information

Under these statutory provisions, the health professional, such as a nurse, has no discretion over whether or not to disclose the information. They are obliged to do so by law.

Scenario 10.5

Disclosure under the provisions of the Road Traffic Act 1988

Under the provisions of the Road Traffic Act 1988, there is a duty to disclose information relating to road traffic offences when asked to do so. In *Hunter v Mann* [1974], a doctor was successfully prosecuted for refusing to disclose information that would have revealed the identity of a person driving dangerously on the grounds that it had been acquired solely through the relationship of doctor and patient, and to divulge it would be a breach of his professional duty of confidence.

The court held that the doctor had been rightly convicted, as the duty imposed by road traffic laws to give information that may lead to the identification of the driver of a vehicle overrides a health professional's duty of confidence to the patient.

Other statutes that require disclosure of information under specific circumstances include:

- the Public Health (Control of Disease) Act 1984 and its regulations, which require a doctor to notify the local authority of the particulars of any person who is suffering from a notifiable disease or food poisoning;
- the National Health Service (Notification of Births) Regulations 1982 (SI 1982/286), which require any person attending a mother to notify the district medical officer of the birth of a child born dead or alive after the twenty-eighth week of pregnancy;
- the Misuse of Drugs (Notification of Supply to Addicts) Regulations 1973, which require a doctor to notify the Home Office of any person he or she considers, or has reasonable grounds to suspect of being, addicted to a notifiable drug.

Disclosing anonymised information

Information is provided by patients in confidence and must be treated as such, as long as it remains capable of identifying the individual it relates to. However, anonymised information is not considered confidential and may be used with few constraints. Information that does not identify an individual directly and that cannot reasonably be used to determine identity is considered to be anonymous information.

Scenario 10.6

Disclosing anonymised information

In *R v Department of Health Ex p. Source Informatics Ltd (No. 1)* [2001], Source Informatics appealed against a policy of the Department of Health, which advised that the practice of GPs and pharmacists selling anonymous prescription details was a breach of confidence. The company argued that the collection of data concerning the prescribing habits of a GP was useful for those seeking to assess prescribing patterns. Although the individual GP, whose consent would be required, was identified, the patient would remain anonymous. The Court of Appeal allowed the appeal as the law was concerned with protecting the right to privacy, but that had not been breached because all the patients' personal details had been expunged.

Effective anonymisation requires more than just the removal of names and addresses. A full postcode, NHS number or even the name of the ward with the date of admission to hospital can be strong identifiers, along with other information such as a date of birth, particularly if looked at in combination with other data items.

Anonymised patient information can be used for a range of purposes, such as audit, effective planning of services, research, education and even inclusion in assignments and journal articles. As Lord Justice Bingham held in *W v Egdell* [1990], if a health professional discloses information about a patient to a newspaper or makes a comment in a journal article or while gossiping with friends, this would be a breach of the duty of confidence unless they took appropriate steps to conceal the identity of the patient.

Disclosing information with appropriate care

The general duty of confidence imposed on registered nurses requires that patient information is kept confidential and must not be disclosed.

However, this duty is not absolute and there will be occasions where confidential information will need to be disclosed.

Given that registered nurses will face sanctions from their employer, professional regulatory body and the law for an unwarranted breach of confidence, it is essential that any disclosure of information is done appropriately within the requirements of the duty owed to the patient.

Where you are unclear as to whether a disclosure of information is justified, you should seek advice from a senior colleague or manager. You must also follow the policies on the use and disclosure of patient information that all NHS establishments are required to have, along with the advice given in *Confidentiality: NHS code of practice* (DH, 2003c). In addition, you must consider the requirements of your *Code* and the law of confidence.

Where a patient has been told that patient information will be recorded and used for the purpose of delivering effective healthcare, you may share information with other members of the clinical team caring for that individual. Disclosure must be restricted to the clinical team only.

Your duty of confidence to the patient generally requires that disclosure of confidential information for purposes other than care and treatment must only be done with the explicit consent of the patient, unless an exception to that duty applies or the information can be disclosed in an anonymised form (NMC, 2008). Anonymous information is information from which all identifying particulars have been removed.

Where you intend to disclose confidential information without the explicit consent of the patient, you will need to consider carefully whether an exception to the general duty of confidence applies.

Human Rights Act 1998

Article 8 of the European Convention on Human Rights may be engaged if the information to be disclosed interferes with the right to respect for private and family life, home and correspondence.

Where the information is disclosed with the consent of the patient, article 8 will not be engaged.

If article 8 is engaged, you will need to demonstrate that disclosure is:

- in accordance with the law;
- in pursuit of a legitimate aim; and
- necessary in a democratic society.

Where the disclosure complies with both the Data Protection Act 1998 and the common law of confidentiality, human rights requirements will generally be satisfied.

Common law of confidence

Under the common law, information is confidential where:

- it has the necessary quality of confidence; and
- it has been communicated in circumstances giving rise to an obligation of confidence.

This would apply to information obtained in the course of the nurse–patient relationship. This information may be shared with other members of the clinical team for purposes relating to care and treatment. Disclosure for any other purpose must only be made with the explicit consent of the patient, unless an exception to the duty arises.

Before disclosing confidential information without consent you will need to consider whether:

- the common law duty has been modified by statute; or
- there is an overriding public interest that justifies disclosure.

Data Protection Act 1998

The Data Protection Act 1998 applies to personal information held on computer or as part of a relevant filing system. This definition would include health records. Under the provisions of the Act a decision to disclose personal health information must be fair and lawful.

To be lawful, the disclosure of personal health information must meet the requirements of the common law duty of confidence and be justified under the requirements of schedules 2 and 3 of the Data Protection Act 1998, which deal with the processing, including disclosure, of personal information and sensitive personal information respectively.

Caldicott Guardians

Each NHS organisation has a guardian of person-based clinical information who oversees the arrangements for its use and sharing.

They ensure that patient-identifiable information is only shared for justified purposes and that only the minimum necessary information is shared in each case.

Every use or flow of patient-identifiable information must be regularly justified and routinely tested against the principles developed in the Caldicott Report.

- Justify the purpose(s) for using confidential information.
- Only use it when absolutely necessary.
- Use the minimum that is required.
- Access should be on a strict need-to-know basis.
- Everyone must understand his or her responsibilities.
- Understand and comply with the law.

The Caldicott Guardian plays a key role in ensuring that the NHS satisfies the highest practical standards for handling patient-identifiable information. The Guardian should actively support work to facilitate and enable information sharing and advise on options for the lawful and ethical processing of information to ensure that such sharing is appropriate.

Activity 10.7

Appropriate disclosure of patient information

Outline how you would ensure the appropriate disclosure of information regarding a patient in your care in the following circumstances:

1. information about the condition of a celebrity admitted to hospital for surgery to the media waiting outside the hospital;
2. information about a large quantity of ecstasy found on a patient admitted to ICU following a road traffic collision;
3. information to managers undertaking an audit of care on the ward;
4. information about a patient's condition to a friend who is enquiring on the telephone;
5. information to a court about a patient's whereabouts on a particular time and day;
6. information about a patient's condition to the doctor in charge of his care.

(Hint: use *Confidentiality: NHS code of practice* (DH, 2003c) as a resource in completing this activity.)

An outline answer is given at the end of the chapter.

In exercising their professional duty, nurses and midwives will both seek and receive information of a confidential nature from their patients. Generally, they will be required to keep this information to themselves and respect the right of the patient not to have their health information disclosed. However, when such information involves, for example, a threat of harm to others, a decision whether or not to disclose that information to others can pose a dilemma.

Nurses have to balance the legal and professional duty to maintain confidentiality against the exceptions to that duty allowing disclosure. While under certain circumstances the courts can require disclosure, it is left largely to nurses to exercise their professional judgement when deciding whether or not to reveal confidential information to others. This leaves them open to a charge of breaching both the professional and legal duty of confidence and risking sanctions that could include losing their job and professional status together with the possibility of damages for the patient. However, the common law and the decisions of the courts have provided guidance for health professionals on what information is confidential, when a duty of confidence exists, and the exceptions to that duty.

Nurses must inform their professional decision making by adhering to the guidance of courts, their code of conduct and the NHS code of practice on confidentiality in resolving the dilemmas that arise from the burden of keeping a confidence. In this way a balance will be reached in maintaining both the patient's right to have their confidences respected and the need to share confidential information where a public interest in protecting others arises.

CHAPTER SUMMARY

- Maintaining the confidentiality of a patient's health information is a fundamental element of professional conduct and ethical practice for all registered nurses.
- Patients pass on sensitive information in confidence and expect you to respect their privacy by ensuring the confidentiality of the information they give.
- A duty of confidence is imposed on nurses to reassure patients that their health information will be respected.
- The duty is imposed by all contracts of employment in the NHS, the NMC's *Code of Professional Conduct* and the law.
- The duty of confidence imposed on nurses is not absolute and is subject to a range of exceptions that justify disclosure.
- Consent from the patient allowing disclosure of confidential information is the starting presumption in law.
- Consent to disclose confidential information to other members of the clinical team may be implied where the patient understands how the information is to be used and has no objections.
- Where a patient refuses to allow information to be disclosed to other health professionals involved in their care, it could result in limited care and treatment.
- There are a number of exceptions allowing disclosure to appropriate sources without the consent of the patient.
- The public interest exception covers a broad range of situations that allow for confidential information to be disclosed without the consent of the patient.
- A statute can modify the duty of confidence owed by a nurse.
- Anonymised information is not considered confidential and may be used with few constraints.

- It is essential that any disclosure of information is done appropriately within the requirements of the duty owed to the patient.
- Each NHS organisation has a guardian of person-based clinical information, known as a Caldicott Guardian, who oversees the arrangements for the use and sharing of clinical information.

Activities: brief outline answers

10.1 Defining confidentiality (page 177)

Confidentiality relates to the duty to maintain confidence and thereby respect the privacy of a patient's health information.

10.2 The need for a duty of confidence (page 178)

Imposing a duty of confidence reassures patients that their personal health information will be treated sensitively and with respect, and will not be disclosed unnecessarily.

10.3 The professional duty of confidence (page 179)

The NMC demands that registered nurses treat a patient's health information as confidential. You are required to inform patients how and why their health information will be shared with those involved in their care. Disclosure must occur where you believe someone to be at risk of harm.

The NMC suggests that disclosure can occur:

- with the consent of the patient;
- without consent where it is necessary in the public interest to protect a person from risk of harm.

Any other disclosure is a matter for a nurse's professional judgement and they will be accountable for that decision. The NMC gives no guidance as to what circumstances might justify disclosure.

10.4 Disclosing information about patients (page 182)

Your list will demonstrate that the duty of confidence is not absolute and a number of exceptions to the duty exists and include disclosure:

- with the consent of the patient;
- for care and treatment purposes;
- when a patient specifically asks you to do so;
- when a patient is incapable of receiving information;
- in cases of suspected abuse of dependent elderly and children;
- in the interests of justice;
- for the public good;
- to protect a third party;
- to prevent or detect a serious crime;
- under statutes that empower the health professional to disclose information;
- under statutes that require information to be disclosed under specific circumstances.

10.5 Share with Care (page 184)

Below are the main findings:

- High level of trust in the NHS to protect patient confidentiality, but low awareness of how the NHS uses patient information.
- People were more concerned about who used the information and whether it was anonymous than how the information would be used.
- People were comfortable with their GP, hospital doctors and emergency services having access to their data, although they reserved the right to limit access to very sensitive information.
- People felt that all others treating them should be allowed access on a 'need to know' basis
- People felt that information released outside the NHS, or used by the NHS for purposes other than treatment, should be anonymised or patient permission sought to use identifiable data.
- Once information was anonymised, a majority were happy not to be asked for consent to share it.
- People differed over how their consent should be obtained for using identifiable information. Some wanted to be asked for a one-off consent; others wanted their consent to be sought each time information was used other than for treatment. Some wanted to be asked every time information was used, including for treatment.

10.6 Breach of confidentiality (page 187)

Gunshot wounds are usually the result of a serious incident and so the police should be told whenever a person has arrived at a hospital with such a wound.

In this case, it would be reasonable to confirm the existence of such a patient without disclosing identifying details, such as the patient's name and address.

Remember that the police are responsible for assessing the risk posed by members of the public who are armed. By knowing of the existence of the patient, the police can consider the risk of a further attack on the patient and also risks to staff, patients and visitors in the A & E department or elsewhere in the hospital.

Once you have confirmed the existence of the patient, the police will usually ask to see him or her. The treatment and care of the patient is your first concern, so do not allow police access to the patient if this will delay or hamper treatment or compromise the patient's recovery.

If a patient's treatment and condition allows them to speak to the police, you should ask the patient whether they are willing to do so. Patients have a right to expect that information about them will be held in confidence by their nurses. This is an important element of a relationship of trust between nurses and patients.

However, if the patient cannot give consent, or says 'no', information can still be disclosed if there are grounds for believing that this is in the public interest or that disclosure is required by law.

Disclosures in the public interest are justified where:

- a failure to disclose information would put the patient, or someone else, at risk of death or serious harm;
- a disclosure may assist in the prevention, detection or prosecution of a serious crime.

Both of these situations might apply in a case where a patient has a gunshot wound.

Remember, if there is any doubt about whether disclosure is justified, the decision to disclose information without consent should be made by, or with the agreement of, the consultant in charge, or the Trust's Caldicott Guardian.

Wherever practicable, patients should be told that a disclosure will be or has been made and the reasons for disclosure must be recorded in the patient's notes.

10.7 Appropriate disclosure of patient information (page 192)

1. Normally, there is no basis for disclosure of confidential and identifiable information about patients to the media. There will be occasions, however, when NHS hospitals and staff are asked for information about individual patients, such as requests for updates on the condition of celebrity patients. Where practicable, the explicit consent of the individual patient concerned must be obtained before disclosing any information about their care and treatment, and that includes their presence in the hospital. Where consent cannot be obtained or is withheld, disclosure will only be justified if it is in the public interest. Where a patient is not competent to make a decision about disclosure, the views of family members should be sought and decisions made in the patient's best interests.

2. The police have no general right of access to health records, but there are statutes that require disclosure to them and some that permit disclosure. The Road Traffic Act 1988 requires disclosure of information that would lead to the identity of a person involved in a road traffic offence and you would be obliged to give this information if asked by a police officer. In the absence of a requirement to disclose, there must be either explicit patient consent or a robust public interest justification. In this case, the public interest in preventing or detecting a serious crime would allow disclosure. Supplying a class A drug such as ecstasy is a serious offence and you would be empowered to disclose the information to the police. Where disclosure is justified, it should be limited to the minimum necessary to meet that purpose and the patient should be informed of the disclosure unless it would defeat the purpose of the investigation, allow a potential criminal to escape or put staff at risk.

3. The evaluation of clinical performance against standards or through comparative analysis, with the aim of informing the management of services, is an essential component of modern healthcare provision and is regarded as a healthcare purpose. Disclosure of information relevant to the audit would be a justified disclosure. Every effort should be made to ensure that patients are aware that audit takes place and that it is essential if the quality of care they receive is to be monitored and improved.

4. Friends often provide valuable help and support to patients, and also act as carers. However, the explicit consent of a competent patient is needed before disclosing information to a friend. The best interests of a patient who is not competent to consent may also warrant disclosure. Where disclosure of information does go ahead, only information essential to a patient's care should be disclosed and patients should be made aware that this is the case.

5. The courts have legal powers to require disclosure of confidential patient information in the interests of justice. However, you need to take care to limit disclosure to the matter required by the court and provide only the precise information requested.

6. Disclosing information to the doctor in charge of the patient's care is a justified disclosure and necessary for the proper treatment of the patient. Patients should be made aware that information about their care will be shared with other members of the clinical team and, where this occurs, the explicit consent of the patient to such a disclosure is not necessary.

Knowledge review

Now that you've worked through the chapter, how would you rate your knowledge of the following topics?

	Good	Adequate	Poor
1. Your duty of confidence to patients.			
2. The exceptions to the general duty of confidence.			
3. How to disclose patient information appropriately.			

Where you are not confident in your knowledge of a topic, what will you do next?

Further reading

Department of Health (DH) (2003) *Confidentiality: NHS code of practice*. London: Department of Health.

NHS Information Authority (2002) *Share with Care: People's views on consent and confidentiality of patient information*. London: NHSIA.

Nursing and Midwifery Council (NMC) (2004a) *Code of Professional Conduct: Standards for conduct, performance and ethics*. London: NMC.

Nursing and Midwifery Council (NMC) (2004b) *Complaints about Unfitness to Practise: A guide for members of the public*. London: NMC.

Useful websites

www.connectingforhealth.nhs.uk NHS information on confidentiality.

www.dh.gov.uk/Informationpolicy/Patientconfidentialityandcaldicottguardians Department of Health information on patient confidentiality and Caldicott Guardians.

www.nhsia.nhs.uk/confidentiality/pages/docs/swc.pdf NHS Information Authority information on confidentiality.

www.nmc-uk.org Nursing and Midwifery Council, which contains guidance on confidentiality issues.

Chapter 11

Health and safety in the workplace

Introduction

Some 1.7 million people are employed by the NHS and ensuring the health and safety of employees is essential to the efficient delivery of healthcare.

Activity 11.1

Risks at work

In a group, list the potential risks to your health and safety that you have encountered during clinical practice. When you have completed that list, make another with the potential hazards faced by patients receiving healthcare.

Now read below for further information.

The Health and Safety Executive (2007) estimate that absence in the NHS costs some £1 billion annually, and the following are the four main causes:

- **Musculoskeletal disorders** – along with stress, these are the biggest cause of sick leave in the NHS, accounting for some 40 per cent. A quarter of all nurses have at some time taken time off as a result of a back injury sustained at work.
- **Stress** – this is a major cause of work-related ill health and sick leave among healthcare employees. Work-related stress accounts for over a third of all new incidences of ill health and each case leads to an average of 30.2 working days lost. A total of 13.8 million working days were lost to work-related stress, depression and anxiety in 2006/7.
- **Violence** – NHS staff and other healthcare workers are four times more likely to experience work-related violence and aggression than other workers. Employers must assess the risk of verbal and physical violence to their employees and take appropriate steps to deal with this risk.
- **Slips and trips** – in 2006/7, 53 per cent (841 of 1,561) of major injuries to employees in the health services were as a result of slips or trips.

Patients are also placed at risk of injury if appropriate safety measures are not taken. The NHS Litigation Authority (2007) estimates that some £500 million is paid annually by the health service in compensation claims and fines for breaching health and safety laws. The cost in human terms can also be high. Mistakes and errors can compromise safety to the point where lives are put at risk and, sadly, fatalities occur. The risk to patients include: medication errors, treatment errors, falls, violence, poorly maintained equipment, human errors, fire and hospital acquired infections.

Scenario 11.1

Patient dropped off at wrong address

Two NHS Trusts were fined a total of £27,500 over the death of a 93-year-old woman, dropped off at the wrong house by an ambulance crew (Hughes and Butler, 2007). The lady, who suffered from dementia, became confused in the unfamiliar surroundings and fell, breaking her leg. She died some five weeks later in hospital.

Nurse left on his own on a ward killed by a patient

A London Trust was fined £28,000 and £14,000 costs at the Old Bailey following a prosecution brought by the Health and Safety Executive, after a nurse was killed by a psychiatric patient (*M2 Presswire*, 2005). The junior member of staff was working alone on the ward without clear procedures and with inadequate measures in place to check on his safety. He suffered multiple injuries that resulted in the loss of his life.

Health and safety law

To prevent the avoidable loss of life and minimise the days lost to absence, the NHS as an employer has a legal duty to comply with the requirements relating to health and safety at work.

The Health and Safety at Work etc. Act 1974 is the basis of health and safety law in the UK, and sets out general duties that:

- employers have towards employees and members of the public using their service;
- employees have to themselves and to each other.

Breaching or failing to comply with these duties are criminal offences.

The employer's general duty is set out in section 2 of the Health and Safety at Work etc. Act 1974 and states that an employer has:

- a duty to ensure *so far as is reasonably practicable*, the health, safety and welfare at work of employees and any others who may be affected by the undertaking . . ..

The legal standard imposed by the 1974 Act is *reasonably practicable* or *so far as is reasonably practicable*. The standard implies a weighing up of the risk against the cost in terms of time, money or trouble of preventing or controlling the risk.

The duty of employees at work is set out in section 7 of the Health and Safety at Work etc. Act 1974, which states that:

- it shall be the duty of every employee while at work:
  - to take reasonable care of their own health and safety and of any other person who may be affected by their acts or omissions;
  - to cooperate with their employer so far as is necessary to enable that employer to meet their requirements with regard to any statutory provisions.

Health and safety duties owed by employees

The Health and Safety at Work etc. Act 1974 places a duty on employees to take reasonable care of their own health and safety. List reasonable measures a registered nurse could take to ensure their health and safety in the course of their work.

An outline answer is given at the end of the chapter.

The duty to report incidents

As well as a duty under the Health and Safety at Work etc. Act 1974, a registered nurse is also under a professional duty to act to identify and minimise risks to patients and clients (NMC, 2008).

A nurse who raises an issue of health and safety with an employer, either directly or through a union, is entitled to protection from dismissal and victimisation under the Public Interest Disclosure Act 1998. Under the Act each NHS employer has a duty to establish a procedure for employees to raise concerns where:

- a criminal offence has been, is being or is likely to be committed; or
- the health or safety of an individual has been, is being or is likely to be endangered.

Scenario 11.3

Concern about infant deaths

A doctor concerned about perinatal mortality rates (stillbirths and deaths of those aged less than one week) in South Tyneside was sacked after highlighting the high infant death rate and the appalling treatment of female patients (*The Journal*, 2006). She ultimately won her case for unfair dismissal and racial discrimination.

Health and safety regulations

The Health and Safety at Work etc. Act 1974 is supplemented by a wide range of secondary legislation in the form of regulations and orders that focus on specific areas of workplace health and safety, such as manual handling. Most of this secondary legislation begins in the form of a European Union Directive that must be implemented in the law of individual member states. The directives aim to harmonise workplace health and safety throughout all countries of the European Union. Table 11.1 lists the main regulations that affect the health service and their employees.

It is essential that employers and staff work together to ensure effective implementation of health and safety measures. This joint approach helps to promote and raise awareness among employers and staff, thereby creating a positive safety culture.

Involving staff in workplace health and safety is a legal requirement under the provisions of the Safety Representatives and Safety Committee Regulations 1977, and the Health and Safety (Consultation with Employees) Regulations 1996, which require staff representatives to:

- consult with and be consulted by employers regarding:
  - the introduction of measures that may affect health and safety;
  - arrangements for appointing competent persons to assess risks;
  - provision of health and safety information and training;
- investigate hazards, accidents and complaints, etc.;
- make representation to the employer on health and safety matters;
- perform workplace inspections;
- be given time off to perform their duties and undertake health and safety training.

Table 11.1: Regulations relating to health and safety in the NHS.

Regulations	Scope
Management of Health and Safety at Work Regulations 1999	Sets out how employers are required to assess risk in all work activities, implement control measures if required, provide information and training, and appoint competent persons.
Manual Handling Operations Regulations 1992	Cover the moving and handling of objects, either by hand or by bodily force.
Control of Substances Hazardous to Health Regulations 2002	Relate to the assessment of hazardous substances and biological agents, and the implementation of appropriate precautions.
Reporting of Injuries, Diseases and Dangerous Occurrences Regulations 1995	Require employers to notify certain types of injury, disease and dangerous occurrences to the Health and Safety Executive.
Personal Protective Equipment at Work Regulations 1992	Cover the provision of suitable and sufficient protective clothing and equipment, such as uniforms and gloves, etc.
Workplace (Health, Safety and Welfare) Regulations 1992	Cover issues such as ventilation, temperature, flooring and workstations, etc.
Health and Safety (Display Screen Equipment) Regulations 1992	Set out requirements for the use of visual display units, workstations, seating, etc.
Provision and Use of Work Equipment Regulations 1998	Cover the safe use and maintenance of equipment, such as hoists.
Health and Safety (First Aid) Regulations 1981	Concern first aid requirements, such as the contents of first aid boxes and the number of trained first aid personnel.
Health and Safety (Safety Signs and Signals) Regulations 1996	Specify the minimum requirements for safety signs at work.
The Fire Precautions (Workplaces) Regulations 1997	Require employers to assess the risk of fire in the workplace.
Hazardous Waste (England and Wales) Regulations 2005	Specify the requirements for the classification, segregation and disposal of waste, including that which is infectious and hazardous.

Managing health and safety

The Health and Safety Executive (2006) requires workplace health and safety to be managed methodically to ensure that risks are minimised. This includes establishing a health and safety policy to provide information on the management of work-related risks. The policy will complement the Trust's policies that relate to specific requirements, such as manual handling and the control of substances hazardous to health.

It also includes demonstrating that health and safety management is organised and functioning by reference to the four Cs.

- **Cooperation:**
  - good safety performance depends on everyone cooperating and safety is everybody's business;
  - there is a legal requirement to consult with staff representatives on health and safety matters.
- **Communication:**
  - consultation with staff safety representatives;
  - performing workplace inspections at regular intervals with written reports available for staff to view;
  - setting up a workplace Safety Committee.
- **Control:**
  - there is a legal requirement to exercise control of health and safety to ensure compliance; if there is failure to comply with an identified safety rule, such as not disposing of clinical waste appropriately, and action is not taken to rectify the situation, both the employer and staff member break the law.
- **Competence:**
  - having the knowledge and skills needed to work without risk to yourself or to others who come into contact with your work;
  - managers must ensure that individuals for whom they are responsible have the appropriate skills and knowledge to work without risk to themselves or to others;
  - competence is a legal requirement imposed on employers through health and safety regulations; training in health and safety measures is a mandatory component of a health service contract.

Activity 11.3

Health and safety training

In a group, discuss which elements of your nursing programme might be considered to be health and safety training, for example fire training, manual handling training, etc. Make a list of the topics covered. Now compare that list with the list of hazards you identified in Activity 11.1. Does the training reflect the hazards you are likely to encounter?

An outline answer is given at the end of the chapter.

The Health and Safety Executive (2006) requirements also include:

- assessment and monitoring of risks:
  - assessment of the risks associated with performing workplace tasks and identification of any workplace precautions and risk control systems that may be required and their successful implementation;

- o   monitoring through inspections and risk assessments;
- review and audit:
  - o   performance must be reviewed against an audit of documentation, such as workplace inspections, risk assessments, accident and incident reports, and attendance on health and safety training courses.

Workplace risk assessments

A risk assessment is the identification of hazards present in the workplace and an estimate of the risk associated with performing a task. A hazard is something that has the potential to cause harm and a risk is the likelihood of that hazard causing an accident or incident.

There is a legal duty to perform risk assessments under the provisions of the Management of Health and Safety at Work Regulations 1999.

Once a hazard has been identified, the likelihood of the risk occurring and the severity of the harm must be considered. The law requires that risks should be reduced *so far as is reasonably practicable*. That means that the degree of risk should be balanced against the time, trouble, cost and physical difficulty of taking measures to avoid it.

On identifying a risk, steps must be taken to minimise it by:

- elimination of the hazard at source; if this is not possible, the hazard must be reduced;
- taking action, if the hazard has to be reduced, to control the risk by introducing workplace precautions, such as alarms, training and information, safety cabinets, ventilation systems, etc.
- putting in place, once workplace precautions have been introduced, a system to monitor compliance with those precautions .

For example, the Control of Substances Hazardous to Health Regulations 2002 seek to control exposure to hazardous substances that arises from work under an employer's control.

The regulations require that exposure of employees to substances hazardous to health is either prevented or, where this is not reasonably practicable, adequately controlled (Control of Substances Hazardous to Health Regulations 2002, Regulation 7(1)).

Employers must, therefore, where reasonably practicable, eliminate completely the use or production of substances hazardous to health in the workplace by changing the method of work, modifying the process or substituting a non-hazardous substance.

Where prevention of exposure to substances hazardous to health is not reasonably practicable, employers must adequately control exposure.

Scenario 11.4

Latex allergy

In *Dugmore v Swansea NHS Trust* [2002], a nurse was awarded £345,000 from her employing Trust for injuries caused by hazardous substances. The nurse was forced to abandon her career due to an allergy to latex and gave up nursing in 1997 after experiencing asthma, skin problems and anaphylactic attacks after exposure to latex.

The Trust was liable because, although they took the step of providing the nurse with latex-free products, other staff on the ward continued to use them and this was enough to trigger an allergic reaction.

Reporting accidents and incidents

Reporting accidents and incidents at work is an essential component of monitoring the effectiveness of health and safety measures, and preventing the recurrence of an incident. In addition to local NHS Trust accident reporting procedures, there is a legal requirement to report certain categories of accidents that occur within the workplace to the Health and Safety Executive under the Reporting of Injuries, Diseases and Dangerous Occurrences Regulations 1995.

Accidents at work are only reportable if they arise out of, or in connection with, work. There are different categories of accidents, including:

- **death or major injuries**: when a member of staff or a patient is killed or suffers a major injury (including injuries sustained as a result of physical violence) while working;
- **injuries that last over three days**: when accidents (including acts of physical violence) result in the injured person being away from work or unable to perform their normal duties for more than three days (including non-working days);
- **diseases**: where a doctor notifies the Trust in writing that an employee is suffering from a disease specified in regulations and linked with a workplace activity; reportable diseases include:
  - occupational dermatitis;
  - occupational asthma or respiratory sensitisation as a result of exposure to chemical substances;
  - infections such as hepatitis, tuberculosis, legionella and tetanus;
  - infection reliably attributable to working with biological agents – exposure to blood or body fluids or any potentially infective material.

Dangerous occurrences

Dangerous occurrences or near misses must also be reported and these are events that may not result in a reportable injury, but have the potential to do significant harm. In the health service reportable occurrences would include:

- collapse, overturning or failure of load-bearing parts of lifts and lifting equipment, such as a hoist;
- explosion, collapse or bursting of any closed vessel or associated pipework, such as an autoclave;
- electrical short-circuit or overload causing fire or explosion;
- explosion or fire causing suspension of normal work for over 24 hours;
- accidental release of any substance that may damage health.

Manual handling

The risk of injury

Musculoskeletal injury, particularly back injury, is one of the most common causes of incapacity among nurses. Secombe and Smith (1996) argue that some 3,600 nurses have to retire each year because of back injuries, with a further 80,000 estimated to have hurt their backs. The Health and Safety Executive shows that, from 1992 to 1995, some 14,000 manual handling accidents were reported in the NHS, with 60 per cent of these involving the handling of patients (Health and Safety Executive, 2002). The National

Audit Office (2003) found that back injury forms a third of all reported injuries in the NHS and claims that only 42 per cent of back injury is actually reported.

Reducing the risk of injury

The Management of Health and Safety at Work Regulations 1999 require employers to make an assessment of the risks to the health and safety of their employees and others they have contact with at work. The regulations further require that protective and preventative measures be put in place to avoid such risks.

The Manual Handling Operations Regulations 1992 deal specifically with the manual handling of loads. Regulation 2(1) defines manual handling as *any transporting or supporting of a load (including the lifting, putting down, pushing, pulling, carrying or moving thereof) by hand or by bodily force.* A load is defined as including *any person and any animal.* It is clear that the scope of the regulations includes the lifting and moving of patients by nursing staff.

Regulation 4 of the 1992 regulations places a duty on employers to avoid hazardous manual handling operations so far as is reasonably practicable. Where this cannot be avoided, the regulation requires an assessment of the manual handling operation and that steps be taken to reduce the risk of injury to the lowest level that is reasonably practicable. Particular consideration should be given to the provision of mechanical assistance, such as hoists, but, where this is not reasonably practicable, employers should explore improvements to the task, the load and the working environment.

Both the general duty to protect the health and safety of employees and the specific duty to reduce risks to health due to the manual handling of loads apply to the NHS, and NHS and Primary Care Trusts have felt the heavy cost of breaching that duty.

Scenario 11.5

Compensation for breaching a statutory duty, causing back injury

In *Knott v Newham Healthcare Trust* [2003], the Court of Appeal upheld an order for the award of £414,000 to a nurse who had injured her back due to the Trust's inadequate arrangements for lifting. The court found that no real steps had been taken to reduce risk of injury and that the Trust was in breach of its statutory duty under the 1992 regulations.

The high cost of awards and, similarly, high legal costs have reinforced the duty of NHS Trusts to protect the health and safety of their employees.

No-lift policies

Activity 11.4

No-lift policies

Before reading this section, read the manual handling the policy of the NHS Trust that you attend for clinical practice. Note the requirements of the policy. Does it allow any form of lifting or moving of patients by manual means?

An outline answer is given at the end of the chapter.

The great majority of Trusts now implement manual handling procedures through a no-lift policy. Tracy and Ruszala (1996) suggest that the no-lift policy is the only means of reducing injury when handling patients. This view is echoed by the RCN, which in its *Code of Practice for Patient Handling* (2002) argues that hazardous manual handling should be eliminated in all but exceptional or life-threatening situations. NHS Trusts and unions representing staff in the health service see the use of a no-lift policy as the key tool in reducing manual handling injuries. Instead of lifting manually, these policies require that the great majority of patient lifting is achieved by mechanical means.

The meaning of 'reasonably practicable'

Despite the liability NHS Trusts face under statutory health and safety provisions, the duty is not absolute. The Health and Safety at Work etc. Act 1974 and its regulations only require the duty to be carried out so far as is reasonably practicable.

The meaning of this phrase was considered by the Court of Appeal in *Edwards v National Coal Board* [1949]. Lord Justice Asquith held that reasonably practicable did not mean physically possible. NHS Trusts are not required to spend all their funds on ensuring the safety of staff. Rather, there is a narrower requirement to balance the likelihood of the risk occurring against the cost in terms of money, time and trouble in averting the risk. In manual handling terms, this has generally been considered to be balancing the risk of injury to staff against the cost and availability of suitable equipment. The rights and preferences of patients were considered secondary to the primary duty of protecting the health and safety of staff. Under no-lift policies, patients would not be moved or lifted if manual handling was assessed as hazardous and suitable equipment was not available.

Activity 11.5

The East Sussex case

To assist you in applying the legal concepts introduced in the next section of the chapter, download and read *R (on the application of A & Others) v East Sussex County Council and Another* [2003] from www.bailii.org/ew/cases/EWHC/Admin/2003/167.html. Then, in a group discuss the facts of the case and whether you agree with the outcome of the case.

An outline answer is given at the end of the chapter.

Since the introduction of the Human Rights Act 1998, however, the High Court has revisited the interpretation of 'reasonably practicable' and now requires the rights of patients to be considered when assessing moving and handling needs (see the box opposite).

Duty to the patient

At common law patients are owed a duty of care that requires that health professionals meet the needs of their patients in accordance with a standard accepted by a responsible body of professional opinion and that stands up to logical analysis (*Bolitho v City and Hackney HA* [1998]). Meeting this duty may require the manual handling of patients even where there is a risk of injury.

Assessing reasonable practicability

R (on the application of A and Others) v East Sussex County Council and Another [2003] EWHC 167 (Admin)

In assessing reasonable practicability the approach is as follows:

a) the possible methods of avoiding or minimising the risk must be considered (in practice the only alternative to manual lifting in a case such as this is likely to be a hoist);

b) the context – the frequency and duration of the manoeuvres – must be considered: the assessment must be based on the pattern of lifting over a period (typically a day), not on an individual lift basis – a particular lift might be done manually if done only once a day but not if required frequently during the day;

c) the risks to the employee in question associated with each of the possible methods must be assessed: there must be an analysis of (1) the likelihood of any injury to the employee, and (2) the severity of any injury to the employee;

d) the impact upon the person, physical, emotional, psychological or social, of each of the possible methods of avoiding manual lifting must be examined: there must be an analysis of:

   i) the physical and mental personality and characteristics of the person and their personality – this necessarily includes the nature and degree of disablement;

   ii) the wishes and feelings of the person: any evinced negative reaction in the nature of dislike, reluctance, fear, refusal or other manifestation of negative attitude is relevant, though not of course determinative;

   iii) the effect upon the person's dignity and rights, including in particular their rights (protected by article 8) to physical and psychological integrity, to respect for their privacy, to develop their personality and to go out into the community and meet others and their right (protected by article 3) to be free from inhuman or degrading treatment.

These considerations will necessarily involve assessing the impact upon the person of carrying out a manoeuvre other than a manual lift in terms of considerations of personal dignity or the amount of respect afforded to their persons, their quality of life generally – their ability to spend their time in activities other than merely performing bodily functions – and, importantly, matters such as their access to the community.

The assessment must be focussed on the particular circumstances of the individual case. Just as context is everything, so the individual assessment is all. Thus, for example:

a) the assessment must take into account the particular person's personal physical and mental characteristics, be 'user focussed' and 'user led' and should be part of the wider care-planning process for that particular individual;

b) there must be an assessment of the particular person's autonomy interests;

c) the assessment must be based on the particular workers involved (not workers in the abstract);

d) the assessment must be based on the pattern of lifting in the particular case.

Scenario 11.6

No compensation for back injury sustained at work

In *King v Sussex Ambulance NHS Trust* [2002], an ambulance man failed in his claim for compensation for an injured back caused by lifting a patient downstairs with a colleague. The Court of Appeal held that the method to be adopted when moving and handling a person had to be appropriate. In judging what is appropriate, the Court requires that account be taken of the circumstances of the case having regard not only to the medical needs of the patient but also their wishes and feelings.

In this case, the Court of Appeal was clear that the Ambulance Trust's duty to the patient required that she be removed to hospital. The limited availability of suitable equipment meant there was little the Trust could do other than allow the manual lifting of the patient down the stairs. This was a hazardous lift and a career-ending injury occurred. The Court held, however, that there was no breach of the Manual Handling Regulations 1992 or negligence on behalf of the Trust.

The common law duty of care requires that a person whose job includes lifting people accepts a greater risk than those whose handling duty is restricted to inanimate objects. When working in healthcare settings the care of patients gives rise to an inherent need for some manual handling to take place.

Human rights issues

A duty to the patient may also arise if rights under the Human Rights Act 1998 are engaged. Article 2 of the Convention places a positive obligation on states to protect life and there would be a duty to manually lift a person away from danger, such as during a building fire, if this were the only method of removal available. No-lift policies that totally prohibit any manual handling would be unlawful as they breach article 2 of the Convention.

Article 3 of the Convention prohibits, without exception, torture and inhuman or degrading treatment. What constitutes inhuman or degrading treatment is a matter of fact and degree in each case.

Scenario 11.7

Degrading treatment of a prisoner

In *Price v United Kingdom* (33394/96) [2001], the injured party was a thalidomide victim with no limbs who had been committed to jail for contempt. In prison she was denied her wheelchair charger and usual assistance in getting to bed or the toilet, which was the same treatment able-bodied prisoners received. The Court held that a breach of article 3 had occurred, as society considers it a basic humane concern to try to ameliorate and compensate for the disabilities faced by a person in the applicant's situation. These compensatory measures come to form part of the disabled person's bodily integrity. Preventing the applicant from bringing her battery charger to her wheelchair when she is sent to prison for one week, or leaving her in unsuitable sleeping conditions so that she has to endure pain and cold, are violations of the right to bodily integrity.

The *Price* scenario illustrates that inhuman and degrading treatment can occur through thoughtless and uncaring actions. To keep a person who is unable to move unaided in conditions where they are very cold or at risk of developing pressure sores because the bed it too hard or unreachable, or where they experience considerable difficulty in attending to their toilet and washing needs, are breaches of article 3. No-lift policies that forbid manual handling in such conditions would again be unlawful.

Human rights obligations may also arise in handling situations under article 8 of the Convention. Unlike the right to life and the right to freedom from inhuman or degrading treatment, rights under article 8 are not absolute but qualified. Under article 8 the countervailing rights of nurses and carers must also be considered.

Everyone is owed a duty of respect for their dignity and, in circumstances where this may be lost, that duty requires action to be taken; for example, if a patient is left too long in a bed or chair and at risk of developing pressure sores, or where a person is left in bodily waste for any appreciable time. A duty of respect for dignity would require, by manual means if necessary, action to restore the individual's dignity. That is not to say that handling a person by mechanical means is inherently undignified. Nor is the respect for dignity absolute. There are circumstances when caring or treating a person requires undignified means to achieve a dignified end. This is recognised by the European Court of Human Rights, which holds that a measure that is convincingly shown to be a therapeutic necessity cannot be a breach of articles 3 or 8 of the Convention (*Herczegfalvy v Austria* (1993)).

A handling situation that gave rise to the patient's right to respect for physiological and psychological integrity would also require respect for the nurse's physiological and psychological integrity. It is clear, therefore, that in circumstances where article 8 rights are engaged a balance needs to be struck between the rights of the patient and the rights of the nurse.

Where the patient has a longer-term disability that requires lifting to ensure social interaction and contact with the community, the Court further held that it would be unlawful to deny the person access on the grounds that mechanical lifting was not available. The Court cited examples, such as failing to take a person out because a power cut meant a hoist could not be used, or restricting time for activities because either a hoist was not available or continence management away from the place of residence required manual handling (*R (on the application of A and Others) v East Sussex County Council and Another* [2003]).

C H A P T E R   S U M M A R Y

- Some 1.7 million people are employed by the NHS and ensuring the health and safety of employees is essential to the efficient delivery of healthcare.
- The Health and Safety Executive estimates that absence in the NHS costs some £1 billion annually.
- Patients are also placed at risk of injury if appropriate safety measures are not taken.
- The basis of health and safety law in the UK is the Health and Safety at Work etc. Act 1974.
- An employer has a duty to ensure, so far as is reasonably practicable, the health, safety and welfare at work of employees and any others who may be affected by the undertaking.
- An employee, while at work, has a duty to take reasonable care of their own health and safety and that of any other person who may be affected by their acts or omissions.

- The Health and Safety at Work etc. Act 1974 is supplemented by a wide range of secondary legislation in the form of regulations that focus on specific areas of workplace health and safety (see Table 11.1, page 202).
- Employers and staff must work together to ensure effective implementation of health and safety measures.
- The Health and Safety Executive requires workplace health and safety to be managed methodically to ensure that risks are minimised.
- There is a legal duty to perform risk assessments under the provisions of the Management of Health and Safety at Work Regulations 1999.
- The Control of Substances Hazardous to Health Regulations 2002 control exposure to hazardous substances that arise out of work.
- It is a legal requirement to report certain accidents that occur in the workplace to the Health and Safety Executive under the Reporting of Injuries, Diseases and Dangerous Occurrences Regulations 1995.
- Musculoskeletal injury, particularly back injury, is one of the most common causes of incapacity among nurses.
- The Manual Handling Operations Regulations 1992 deal specifically with the manual handling of loads.
- There will be circumstances where the risk to the patient, if not lifted, will override the nurse's ordinary health and safety concerns, even where manual handling would be considered hazardous.
- In the case of hazardous handling situations, manual handling will be the exception rather than the rule.

Activities: brief outline answers

11.1 Risks at work (page 199)

Nurses
Your list should include:
- musculoskeletal disorders;
- stress;
- violence;
- slips and trips.

Patients
Your list should include:
- medication errors;
- treatment errors;
- falls;
- violence;
- poorly maintained equipment;
- human error;
- fire;
- hospital acquired infections.

11.2 Health and safety duties owed by employees (page 200)

Your list will include:
- wearing appropriate personal protective equipment;
- regular attendance at health and safety training;
- complying with health and safety policies for the NHS Trust;
- reporting hazards and incidents promptly;

- seeking assistance when necessary;
- working with the employer to improve health and safety.

11.3 Health and safety training (page 203)

Your list detailing the training you have received should coincide with the main hazards faced by NHS staff as identified by the Health and Safety Executive. Training should therefore include moving and handling loads, fire training, prevention of violence, and breakaway training and managing stress.

11.4 No-lift policies (page 206)

To be lawful, a no-lift policy should allow lifting or moving by manual means where the life of a patient is at risk, where a patient is likely to face inhuman or degrading treatment or where it is necessary to maintain dignity or contact with the community.

11.5 The East Sussex case (page 207)

The case is an interesting analysis of health and safety in nursing and of no-lift policies in particular. It does raise questions about the rights of the nurse compared to the rights of the patient. Should you be required to put yourself at risk of injury to preserve the human rights of a patient?

Knowledge review

Now that you've worked through the chapter, how would you rate your knowledge of the following topics?

	Good	Adequate	Poor
1. The relationship between nursing and health and safety law.			
2. The general duties owed by employers and employees under the Health and Safety at Work etc. Act 1974.			
3. The regulations governing specific health and safety requirements in the NHS.			
4. The process of health and safety management.			
5. The requirements for the safe handling of loads.			
6. The term 'reasonably practicable' in relation to manual handling.			

Where you are not confident in your knowledge of a topic, what will you do next?

Further reading

National Audit Office (2003) *A Safer Place to Work: Improving the management of health and safety risks to staff in NHS Trusts* (House of Commons Papers). London: NAO.

Useful website

www.hse.gov.uk Health and Safety Executive.

References

Anderson, M (2003) One flew over the psychiatric unit: mental illness and the media. *Journal of Psychiatric and Mental Health Nursing,* 10(3): 297.

Attewill, F (2007) Jehovah's Witness mother dies after refusing blood transfusion. *The Guardian,* 5 May.

Audit Commission (2002) *Setting the Record Straight.* London: Audit Commission.

Bainham, A (1990) *Children: The new law.* London: Family Law.

Beauchamp, T and Childress, J (1989) *Principles of Biomedical Ethics.* Oxford: Oxford University Press.

Brindley, M (2003) Doctors find code writing is best way to treat patients. *The Western Mail,* 19 August, p8.

Butler-Sloss, E (2003) *Are We Failing the Family? Human rights, children and the meaning of family in the 21st century.* London: Department for Constitutional Affairs.

Council of Europe (1950) *European Convention on Fundamental Human Rights and Freedoms.* Rome: Council of Europe.

Creighton, S (2006) *Child Protection Statistics.* London: NSPCC Research Department.

Crown Prosecution Service (2004) *Code for Crown Prosecutors.* London: CPS.

David Bennett Inquiry (2003) *Report of an Independent Inquiry into the Death of David Bennett under HSG (94) 27 by Sir John Blofield, Chair.* Cambridge: Norfolk, Suffolk and Cambridge Strategic Health Authority.

Davies, N (1992) *Murder on Ward Four.* London: Chatto.

Department for Constitutional Affairs (2007) *Mental Capacity Act 2005 Code of Practice.* London: The Stationery Office.

Department of Health (DH) (1997) *Children Act 1989: Guidance and regulations.* London: HMSO.

Department of Health (DH) (1999a) *Code of Practice to the Mental Health Act 1983.* London: HMSO.

Department of Health (DH) (1999b) *Working Together to Safeguard Children.* London: The Stationery Office.

Department of Health (DH) (2002) *No Secrets: Guidance on developing and implementing multi-agency policies and procedures to protect vulnerable adults from abuse.* London: The Stationery Office.

Department of Health (DH) (2003a) *The Investigation of Events that Followed the Death of Cyril Mark Isaacs.* London: The Stationery Office.

Department of Health (DH) (2003b) *The Victoria Climbié Inquiry (Lord Laming CM 5730).* London: The Stationery Office.

Department of Health (DH) (2003c) *Confidentiality: NHS code of practice.* London: Department of Health.

Department of Health (DH) (2003d) *Every Child Matters (Cm 5860)*. London: The Stationery Office.

Department of Health (2004) *Independent Investigation Into How The NHS Handled Allegations About the Conduct of Clifford Ayling (Chair: The Honourable Mrs Justice Pauffley)* (Cmd 6298). London: Department of Health.

Dimond, B (2006) What is the law if a patient refuses treatment based on the nurse's race? *British Journal of Nursing* 15(19): 1077–8.

Disability Rights Commission (2003) *Conditions Imposed on a Wheelchair User's Attendance at an International Rugby Union Ground* (DRC 00353). London: DRC.

Edwards, S (1996) *Nursing Ethics: A principle based approach.* London: Palgrave.

Equality and Human Rights Commission (2007) *Interim Business Plan 2007–08.* London: EHR.

European Commission (2007) *Developing a Community Framework for Safe, High Quality and Efficient Health Services.* Brussels: European Commission.

Evening Gazette (2006) Struck off. 31 January, p5.

Gillon, R (1994) Medical ethics: four principles plus attention to scope. *BMJ* 309: 184.

Hampshire and Isle of Wight Counter Fraud Team (2007) Student midwife starts jail sentence. *Fraud Matters*, June, p1.

Health and Safety Executive (2002) *Health and Safety Statistics.* London: HSE.

Health and Safety Executive (2006) *Five Steps to Risk Assessment.* London: HSE.

Health and Safety Executive (2007) *Health and Safety in Health and Social Care Services.* London: HSE.

HM Government (2006) *Working Together to Safeguard Children.* London: The Stationery Office.

Hughes, G and Butler, C (2007) Ambulances 'must improve to stop another tragedy'; report paints damning picture. *Daily Post*, 29 January, p5.

The Journal (2006) Trust faces £2 million legal bill. 17 May, p15.

Kennedy, I and Grubb, A (1998) *Principles of Medical Law.* Oxford: Oxford University Press.

Kirby, D (2004) Care boss and a box of teeth. *Manchester Evening News*, 16 March, p22.

Law Commission (1993) *Consultation Paper 130: Mentally Incapacitated and Other Vulnerable Adults: Public law protection.* London: The Stationery Office.

Lewis, F and Batey, M (1982) Clarifying autonomy and accountability in nursing services. *Journal of Nursing Administration* 12(9): 13–18

Mack, T (2006) Taxi driver refused to give lift to blind man. *Leicester Mercury*, 18 December, p6.

Marsh, B and Narain, J (2003) Patient died because of GP's bad handwriting. *Daily Mail*, 4 February, p4.

Ministry of Justice (2008) *Deprivation of Liberty: Code of Practice to supplement the main Mental Capacity Act 2005 Code of Practice.* London: TSO.

M2 Presswire (2005) Fine following death of nurse at NHS mental health trust. 5 May.

Nathan, H (1957) *Medical Negligence.* London: Butterworths.

National Audit Office (2003) *A Safer Place to Work.* London: NAO.

National Health Service (NHS) Information Authority (2002) *Share with Care: People's views on consent and confidentiality of patient information.* London: NHSIA.

National Health Service (NHS) Litigation Authority (2007) *Annual Report and Accounts 2007* (HC 908). London: The Stationery Office.

Nazroo, J (2001) *Ethnicity, Class and Health.* London: Policy Studies Institute.

Northern Echo (2006) Staff looked at Sir Bobby's records. 25 November, p12.

Nursing and Midwifery Council (NMC) (2002) Coventry nurse struck off for failing to keep proper records (NMC Press Statement 224/02). London: NMC.

Nursing and Midwifery Council (NMC) (2004a) *Code of Professional Conduct: Standards for conduct, performance and ethics.* London: NMC.

Nursing and Midwifery Council (NMC) (2004b) *Complaints about Unfitness to Practise: A guide for members of the public.* London: NMC.

Nursing and Midwifery Council (NMC) (2004c) *Standards of Proficiency for Pre-registration Nursing Education.* London: NMC.

Nursing and Midwifery Council (NMC) (2006) *Case Study: Maladministration of medicines.* London: NMC.

Nursing and Midwifery Council (NMC) (2007) *NMC Record Keeping Guidance.* London: NMC.

Nursing and Midwifery Council (NMC) (2008) *The Code: Standards of conduct, performance and ethics for nurses and midwives.* London: NMC.

Payne, S (2004) Black nurse told not to treat white baby awarded £20,000. *The Daily Telegraph,* 18 May, p11.

Rideout, RW (1983) *Principles of Labour Law.* London: Sweet and Maxwell.

Royal College of Nursing (RCN) (2002) *Code of Practice for Patient Handling.* London: RCN.

Savage, J and Moore, L (2004) *Interpreting Accountability: An ethnographic study of practice nurses, accountability and multidisciplinary team decision-making in the context of clinical governance.* London: Royal College of Nursing.

Secombe, I and Smith, G (1996) Voting with their feet. *Nursing Standard* 11(1): 22–3.

Sinclair, K (2003) Two nurses convicted of causing patient's death. *The Herald* (Glasgow), 28 October, p9.

Stephen Lawrence Enquiry (1999) *Report of an Inquiry into the Murder of Stephen Lawrence by Sir William Macpherson of Cluny Presented to Parliament by the Home Secretary February 1999* (Cmd 4262-I). London: Home Office.

This is Worcestershire (2004) Care assistant loses unfair sacking claim. 17 June, p3.

Thompson, I, Melia, K and Boyd, K (2000) *Nursing Ethics.* London: Churchill Livingstone.

Tracy, M and Ruszala, S (1996) *Introducing a Safer Handling Policy.* London: National Back Pain Association.

United Nations Children's Fund (2003) *A League Table of Child Maltreatment Deaths in Rich Nations* (Innocenti Report Card No. 5). Florence: Unicef.

Unsworth, C (1987) *The Politics of Mental Health Legislation.* Oxford: Clarendon Press.

Western Daily Press (2006) Sacked on the spot for being diabetic. 9 February, p6.

Wright, O (2003) Doctors taught art of writing clearer notes. *The Times* (London), p10.

Index